MCQs on Community Health Nursing

MCQs on Community Health Nursing

Nirmallya Chatterjee MSc (N), MSc (Psycho and Counseling)
Lecturer
Community Health Nursing
BM Birla College of Nursing
Kolkata, West Bengal

JAYPEE
JAYPEE BROTHERS MEDICAL PUBLISHERS
The Health Sciences Publisher
New Delhi | London

Jaypee Brothers Medical Publishers (P) Ltd

Headquarters
EMCA House
23/23-B, Ansari Road, Daryaganj
New Delhi 110 002, India
Landline: +91-11-23272143, +91-11-23272703
+91-11-23282021, +91-11-23245672
E-mail: jaypee@jaypeebrothers.com

Corporate Office
4838/24, Ansari Road, Daryaganj
New Delhi 110 002, India
Phone: +91-11-43574357
Fax: +91-11-43574314
E-mail: jaypee@jaypeebrothers.com

Overseas Office
J.P. Medical Ltd
83 Victoria Street, London
SW1H 0HW (UK)
Phone: +44 20 3170 8910
E-mail: info@jpmedpub.com

EU GPSR Authorised Representative
Logos Europe, 9 rue Nicolas Poussin
17000, La Rochelle, France
Phone: +33 (0) 6 67 93 73 78
E-mail: contact@logoseurope.eu

Website: www.jaypeebrothers.com
Website: www.jaypeedigital.com

Website: www.jaypeebrothers.com
Website: www.jaypeedigital.com

Inquiries for bulk sales may be solicited at: jaypee@jaypeebrothers.com

MCQs on Community Health Nursing

First Edition: **2014**

Reprint: **2026**

ISBN 978-93-5152-226-3

Printed at: Samrat Offset Pvt. Ltd.

Preface

According to World Health Organization, the special field of nursing that combines the skills of nursing is public health and some phases of social assistance and functions as part of the total public health program for the promotion of health, the improvement of the conditions in the social and physical environment, rehabilitation of illness and disability.

This book is completely based on the recent information about the community health, epidemiology, all communicable and noncommunicable diseases, demography and family planning, maternal and child health, health and nutrition, environmental condition, public health policies, social behavioral and communication science, statistics related to community health nursing practice.

At the end of the book, there are few pictorial appendices for diagnosing some disease condition as well as the usability of the herbs and vegetables easily available in the community which are in terms very useful to prevent some of the physical ailments. The book is a pocket-sized yet I hope that this book will help the nursing students to attend their viva voce during their practical examination.

Nirmallya Chatterjee

Acknowledgments

I am grateful to many who encouraged and supported me with their time and encouragement throughout including BM Birla College of Nursing Administrators.

My mother, Mrs Uma Chatterjee and father, Late Mr Kalyan Chatterjee.

Specially to my students who compelled me to write this book.

Also my warmest appreciation goes to M/s Jaypee Brothers Medical Publishers (P) Ltd., New Delhi, for giving the chance to turn my vision into reality.

Contents

1. Concepts of Health and Disease 1
2. Epidemiology: Principles and Practice 10
3. Epidemiology of Communicable Diseases 29
4. Epidemiology of Noncommunicable Diseases 92
5. Demography and Family Health 102
6. Maternal and Child Health 109
7. Nutrition in Public Health 117
8. Physical and Biological Environmental Effect on Health 131
9. Public Health Administration and Community Health Care in India 144
10. Health Systems and Policies 163
11. Social, Behavioral and Communication Sciences 172
12. Statistics 181

Appendix I *203*

Appendix II *215*

Bibliography *221*

1 Concepts of Health and Disease

Q. 1. ***Human diseases are due to bad clouds was a part of which theory?***

i. Supernatural causes
ii. Miasma theory
iii. Germ theory
iv. Epidemiological trial

Q. 2. ***The theory of "epidemiological web of causation" was forwarded by:***

i. Robert Koch and Louis Pasteur
ii. McMahon and colleagues
iii. Henle-Koch
iv. John Stuart Mill

Q. 3. ***The time interval that elapses between the point when "sufficient cause" becomes operative to the point when the first pathological changes of disease start in the body is:***

i. Generation time
ii. Induction period
iii. Latent period
iv. Lag phase

Q. 4. ***Which of the following dimensions is not included in the WHO definition of health?***

i. Physical well-being
ii. Occupational well-being
iii. Mental well-being
iv. Social well-being

Q. 5. ***Physical quality of life index (PQLI) includes the following parameters:***

i. IMR (infant mortality rate), per capita calorie intake and life expectancy
ii. IMR, life expectancy at 1 year and literacy

iii. IMR, MMR (maternal mortality rate) and life expectancy
iv. IMR, life expectancy at birth and literacy

Q. 6. ***A good indicator of the availability, utilization and effectiveness of health care services in a country is:***

i. Maternal mortality rate
ii. Hospital bed occupancy rate
iii. Infant mortality rate
iv. Disability adjusted life years

Q. 7. ***'The systematic study of the means by which biomedical and other relevant knowledge is brought to bear on the health of individuals and communities under a given set of conditions' is the definition given to:***

i. Biomedical research
ii. Health systems research
iii. Intersectoral research
iv. Operations research

Q. 8. ***Sickness is a state of:***

i. Social dysfunction
ii. Subjective state of a person feeling unwell
iii. Impaired physiological function
iv. Impaired psychological function

Q. 9. ***Disease causation is best explained by:***

i. Theory of one-to-one relationship between causal agent and disease
ii. Supernatural theory of disease
iii. Empirical theory of disease causation
iv. Multifactorial theory of disease causation

Q. 10. ***'Course of a disease process without any intervention' is the definition of:***

i. Spectrum of disease
ii. Epidemiology of disease
iii. Natural history of disease
iv. Iceberg phenomenon

Q. 11. ***In the natural history of disease, the pathogenesis phase is deemed to start upon:***

i. Entry of the disease agent in the human host
ii. Interaction between agent, host and environmental factors

iii. Appearance of signs and symptoms
iv. Appearance of complications

Q. 12. ***The term 'disease control' employs all of the following except:***

i. Reducing the complications
ii. Reducing the risk of further transmission
iii. Reducing the incidence of disease
iv. Reducing the prevalence of the disease

Q. 13. ***Morbidity in a community can best be estimated by:***

i. Active surveillance
ii. Sentinel surveillance
iii. Passive surveillance
iv. Monitoring

Q. 14. ***Sentinel surveillance is employed to:***

i. Establish natural history of disease
ii. Detect the total number of cases of a disease in a community
iii. Detect the missing/hidden cases in a community
iv. Plan intervention

Q. 15. ***Education and motivation for healthy lifestyle is:***

i. Primordial prevention
ii. Secondary prevention
iii. Health promotion
iv. Specific protection

Q. 16. ***Disability limitation is part of:***

i. Primordial prevention
ii. Primary prevention
iii. Secondary prevention
iv. Tertiary prevention

Q. 17. ***Which level of prevention is applicable for implementation in a population without any risk factors?***

i. Primordial prevention
ii. Primary prevention
iii. Secondary prevention
iv. Tertiary prevention

Q. 18. ***Use of chemoprophylactic drugs to protect against malaria is:***

i. Primordial prevention
ii. Primary prevention
iii. Secondary prevention
iv. Tertiary prevention

Q. 19. ***Measures that can be applied at the stage of early, discernible disease include:***

i. Primordial and primary prevention
ii. Primary and secondary prevention
iii. Secondary and tertiary prevention
iv. Primary, secondary and tertiary prevention

Q. 20. ***Which of the following is not primary prevention?***

i. Pulse polio immunization
ii. Vitamin A supplementation
iii. Breast self-examination for tumor
iv. Isoniazid (INH) to a baby breast-fed by a sputum positive tubercular mother

Q. 21. ***Which of the following is not tertiary prevention?***

i. Total mastectomy for breast cancer
ii. Tendon transplant in leprosy
iii. Physiotherapy in residual poliomyelitis
iv. Provision of spectacles for refractive errors

Q. 22. ***Any restriction or lack of ability to perform an activity in the manner or within the range considered normal for a human being is called:***

i. Impairment
ii. Handicap
iii. Disability
iv. Disease

Q. 23. ***Choose the correct sequence in order of occurrence.***

i. Disease→disability→impairment→handicap
ii. Disease→impairment→handicap→disability
iii. Handicap→disease→impairment→disability
iv. Disease→impairment→disability→handicap

Q. 24. ***Alma-Ata declaration was held in:***

i. 1976
ii. 1977

iii. 1978
iv. 1980

Q. 25. ***The Global Strategy for Health for all by the year 2000 (HFA2000) set the following guiding targets to be achieved by year 2000 except:***

i. Life expectancy at birth above 60 years
ii. Infant mortality rate below 50 per 1000 live births
iii. Under-5 mortality rate below 70 per 1000 live births
iv. MMR below 301/lakh

Q. 26. ***The Millennium Development Goals which were derive out of the eight chapters of the United Nations Millennium Declaration was held in the year:***

i. 1999
ii. 1978
iii. 2000
iv. 2001

Q. 27. ***The "All India Institute of Hygiene and Public Health" is located in:***

i. Delhi
ii. Mumbai
iii. Kolkata
iv. Chennai

Q. 28. ***The golden age of public health is:***

i. 1790–1840
ii. 1840–1880
iii. 1880–1970
iv. 1970–2000

Q. 29. ***The global adult literacy rate is:***

i. 70.2%
ii. 78.4%
iii. 80.9%
iv. 62.9%

Q. 30. ***Globally, the percentage of population having access to improved sanitation is:***

i. 60
ii. 80
iii. 86
iv. 72

Answer with explanation

Ans. 1. ii. Miasma theory was illustrated by epidemiologists like William Farr which postulated that human diseases are due to bad clouds which are more dense at lower altitudes and hence diseases are more common among people who live nearer to the earth or sea level; in fact Farr tried to prove this by data taken from London cholera epidemic during midnineteenth century.

Ans. 2. ii. McMahon and colleagues.

Ans. 3. ii. Induction period.

Ans. 4. ii. WHO in the preamble to its constitution defines health as 'health is a state of complete physical, mental and social well-being and not merely an absence of disease or infirmity'. In recent years, it has been amplified to include spiritual well-being and ability to lead a socially and economically productive life.

Ans. 5. ii. In a scale of 0–100, the PQLI is an average of three indicators, i.e. infant mortality rate, life expectancy at 1 year and literacy. It is notable that PQLI does not take GNP into consideration.

Ans. 6. iii. IMR is considers as the sensitive index of health service as it reflex maternal care, perinatal care, child raring practice, nutritional status and the socio-economic condition in which people live as well as availability, effectiveness and utilization of health care services.

Ans. 7. ii. Health systems research deals with all aspects of management of health services including prioritization of health problems, planning, management, logistics and delivery of health care services as well as cost benefit and cost effectiveness of health care systems and biomedical research.

Ans. 8. i. Susser's tentnology suggests that sickness is a state of social dysfunction, i.e. a role an individual assumes when ill; illness is a subjective state of a person who feels that he is not well whereas disease is a physiological/psychological dysfunction.

Ans. 9. iv. Germ theory of disease, i.e. one-to-one relationship between causal agents (microbes) and disease held ground throughout the 19th and early part of the 20th century. It demolished supernatural theory of disease. The modern concept of disease causation is "Web of Causation" suggested by McMahon and Pugg. It largely dwells on the multifactorial causation as well as the well-known 'epidemiological triad of disease' being the result of interplay of agent, host and environmental factors.

Ans. 10. iii. Each disease has its own unique natural history in individuals which is not necessarily same in all the individuals. On the other hand, spectrum of disease and iceberg phenomenon are related to behavior of the disease in the community.

Ans. 11. i. Customarily, natural history of disease is described to have two phases, i.e. prepathogenesis and pathogenesis. Prepathogenesis phase is interaction between agent, host and environment, the agent yet to gain entry into the human body. All other states listed above are related to period of pathogenesis. This understanding of natural history in relation to each disease is the key to plan interventions.

Ans. 12. iv. In disease control, the agent continues to persist in the community though below the critical level where it ceases to be a public health problem. A state of equilibrium is established between the disease agent, host and environment so that new cases cease to occur. Most control activities focus on primary or secondary prevention or both.

Ans. 13. i. Active surveillance implies activities designed to aggressively look for cases of a disease in the community. It thus reveals true pattern of morbidity, whereas in passive surveillance only those cases get counted which report to the health facility with specific symptoms of that disease. Thus, many cases will go unrecorded. Sentinel surveillance on the other hand, is the best way to find out hidden cases. In this, all patients reporting to a health facility (sentinel facility) get checked for a particular disease even if they have reported for other morbidities.

Ans. 14. iii. Detect the missing/hidden cases in a community.

Ans. 15. iii. Health promotion.

Ans. 16. iv. Tertiary prevention.

Ans. 17. i. Although there is no strict delineation between primordial and primary prevention yet primordial prevention can be considered as primary prevention in its purest sense. It is a series of actions applied to entire communities or populations designed to prevent occurrence of diseases whose risk factors have not yet appeared in the communities, e.g. discouraging children from adopting unhealthy lifestyles like smoking, junk foods, sedentary lifestyle, etc. with the long-term aim of preventing obesity, hypertension, coronary heart disease, etc.

It is achieved through individual as well as mass health education. As opposed to this, primary prevention is designed to prevent the onset of disease prior to its occurrence with risk factors already existing, e.g. diet supplements for pregnant or lactating mothers, healthful housing, etc.

Ans. 18. ii. Primary prevention.

Ans. 19. iii. Secondary and tertiary prevention.

Ans. 20. iii. Breast self-examination is a classical example of action taken for early diagnosis and treatment, hence it is secondary prevention. The modes of intervention in primary prevention include:

firstly, health promotion, viz. proper nutrition, environmental sanitation, health education and correct lifestyle; secondly, it includes specific protection, viz. immunization, vitamin A supplementation, chemoprophylaxis, etc.

Ans. 21. i. Total mastectomy for breast tumor is a part of curative therapy, hence it is secondary prevention. In case of tertiary prevention, all actions are designed to limit the disability or provide vocational, social, medical or psychological rehabilitation.

Ans. 22. iii. Disability is the consequence of an impairment whereby the affected person may be unable to carry out certain activities commensurate with his/her age, sex, etc. 'Impairment' is defined as any loss or abnormality of psychological, physiological or anatomical structure or function. On the other hand, a handicap is the disadvantage a person suffers so that he/she is not able to discharge his/her due role in the society. Disease refers to any departure from a healthy condition in an organism.

Ans. 23. iv. In the order of occurrence the process is initiated by disease which leads to impairment, which, if not handled properly, leads to disability.

Handicap results as a consequence of disability. The above terms can be explained as follows:

Accident of soldier (disease)—Amputation of foot (impairment)—Inability to walk (disability)→ Unemployment as a soldier (handicap).

Ans. 24. iii. 1978.

Ans. 25. iv. MMR below 301/lakh.

Ans. 26. iii. 2000.

Ans. 27. iii. Kolkata.

Ans. 28. iii. 1880–1970.

Ans. 29. ii. 78.4%.

Ans. 30. i. 60.

2 Epidemiology: Principles and Practice

Q.1. ***Epidemiology is*:**

i. Branch of medical science which treats epidemics
ii. Science of the mass phenomenon of infectious diseases
iii. Study of disease, any disease, as a mass phenomenon
iv. Study of distribution and determinants of disease frequency in masses
v. All of the above

Q.2. ***In a community, an increase in new cases of a particular disease is due to*:**

i. Increase in incidence rate
ii. Increase in prevalence rate
iii. Both of the above
iv. None of the above

Q.3. ***The most effective tool for measuring incidence of a disease in a community is*:**

i. Case control study
ii. Cohort study
iii. Cross-sectional study
iv. Cross over study

Q.4. ***In a given population, prevalence of a disease can be rapidly determined by*:**

i. Case control study
ii. Cross over study
iii. Cross-sectional study
iv. Double blind study

Q.5. ***If a drug prevents mortality but does not affect cure, then which of the following will be true*:**

i. Incidence will decrease

ii. Incidence will increase
iii. Prevalence will decrease
iv. Prevalence will increase

Q.6. ***In a case control study of smoking and lung cancer, which of the following can be a possible conclusion?***

i. Smoking is a cause of lung cancer
ii. Lung cancer is commoner in smokers than non-smokers
iii. If smoking is stopped, the number of cases of lung cancer will decrease
iv. Smoking is associated with lung cancer

Q.7. ***The ratio between incidence of disease among exposed persons and incidence among nonexposed persons is commonly known as:***

i. Odds ratio
ii. Relative risk
iii. Attributable risk
iv. Population attributable risk

Q.8. ***The number of patients required in a clinical trial to treat a specific disease increases as:***

i. The incidence of the disease decreases
ii. The size of the expected treatment effect increases
iii. The drop-out rate increases
iv. The significance level increases

Q.9. ***The purpose of a double blind study is to:***

i. Avoid subject bias
ii. Avoid observer bias and sampling variation
iii. Reduce the effects of sampling variation
iv. Avoid subject bias and sampling variation

Q.10. ***A clinically manifest disease of man or animal resulting from an infection is called:***

i. Infectious disease
ii. Contagious disease
iii. Iatrogenic disease
iv. Nosocomial disease

Q.11. ***All of the following are true about subclinical cases except:***

i. Responsible for immunity in adults to a variety of infections
ii. Can be detected only by laboratory tests
iii. Host does not shed the infectious agent
iv. Play a significant role in maintaining endemicity (chain of infection) in the community

Q.12. ***Subclinical infection is seen in all except:***

i. Hepatitis B
ii. Measles
iii. Poliomyelitis
iv. Japanese encephalitis

Q.13. ***Latent infection is not seen in:***

i. Ancylostomiasis
ii. Brill-Zinsser disease
iii. Japanese encephalitis
iv. Herpes simplex

Q.14. ***Nature and extent of primary response to an antigen depends on:***

i. Nature and dose of antigen
ii. Route of administration
iii. Nutritional status of host
iv. All of the above

Q.15. ***All of the following are characteristics of a 'secondary immune response' except:***

i. Antibody production is more abundant
ii. Antibodies have greater capacity to bind with the antigen
iii. Response lasts for a shorter period
iv. Shorter latent period

Q.16. ***The Expanded Program of Immunization (EPI) was started in India in 1978. It included all of the following vaccines except:***

i. BCG
ii. Measles
iii. Typhoid
iv. DPT

Q.17. ***The process, which destroys all microbial life including spores is known as:***

i. Disinfection
ii. Antisepsis
iii. Deodorization
iv. Sterilization

Q.18. ***Which of the following is not a complete sterilizing agent?***

i. Glutaraldehyde
ii. Absolute alcohol
iii. Hydrogen peroxide
iv. Sodium hypochlorite

Q.19. ***If a screening test is used in series twice, which parameter will increase?***

i. Sensitivity
ii. Positive predictive value
iii. Specificity
iv. None of the above

Q.20. ***For ruling out of the disease which test is preferred?***

i. Highly sensitive test
ii. Low sensitive test
iii. Highly specific test
iv. None of the above

Q.21. ***Which of the following is a fixed parameter of screening test?***

i. Sensitivity
ii. Negative predictive value
iii. Positive predictive value
iv. None of the above

Q.22. ***Predictive value of screening test depends on:***

i. Prevalence
ii. Sensitivity
iii. Health worker
iv. None of the above

Q.23. ***The following consideration is not required to be taken while doing a screening program:***

i. The disease should be a public health problem

ii. The disease should be vaccine preventable
iii. There should be an acceptable and effective treatment
iv. Facilities for confirming the diagnosis and for treatment should be available

Q.24. ***Among the following, which type of survey provides an exact estimate of incidence:***

i. Hospital-based survey
ii. Hybrid survey
iii. Cross-sectional survey
iv. Longitudinal survey

Q.25. ***What type of survey is a hybrid survey?***

i. Repeated cross-sectional survey
ii. Hospital-based survey
iii. Community-based survey
iv. Longitudinal surveys

Q.26. ***A list of all the sampling units (persons or households) in the actual study population is known as the:***

i. Cluster sample
ii. Sampling ratio
iii. Sampling rate
iv. Sampling frame

Q.27. ***The large collection of humanity to which the findings of the survey will be generalized is called:***

i. Study population
ii. Sample population
iii. Universe
iv. Common population

Q.28. ***All of the following are important ethical issues that need to be addressed in a proposed survey, except:***

i. Provision of cash benefit
ii. Provision of health care benefit
iii. Confidentiality
iv. Informed consent

Q.29. ***While organizing and executing the field work in conduct of a epidemiological survey, in which method is a "line of flow" (i.e. creation of different stations for different activities) needed to be made:***

i. Home visit method
ii. Work place method
iii. Survey center method
iv. Multicentric method

Q.30. ***The primary target audience towards whom the findings of a survey are to be commensurate with, and towards whom the report language is to be directed at, would include all of the following groups of people, except:***

i. Local administrators
ii. Local political leaders
iii. Local health care providers
iv. Urban elite

Q.31. ***All of the following are the uses of surveillance except:***

i. To develop epidemiologic research questions
ii. To develop registries
iii. To test epidemiologic hypothesis
iv. To study the natural history of disease

Q.32. ***For what two issues should a surveillance system be periodically evaluated at the functional level:***

i. Incidence and prevalence
ii. Relevance and repeatability
iii. Completeness and accuracy
iv. Sensitivity and specificity

Q.33. ***Health workers going into the community in search of cases is an example of:***

i. Sentinel surveillance
ii. Passive surveillance
iii. Mass surveillance
iv. Active surveillance

Q.34. ***Prior to setting up a surveillance system, careful consideration needs to be given to all the following aspects of the disease/ health event in question, except:***

i. Economic impact
ii. Public interest
iii. Academic interest
iv. Preventability

Q.35. ***During data analysis (inferential statistics), analytic procedures usually are based on comparing the current incidence against the*:**

i. Mean and standard deviation
ii. Upper and lower control limits
iii. Standard error of mean and proportion
iv. Coefficient of variation

Q.36. ***For long-term secular trends and cyclical trends, the most simple and suitable method is to present a*:**

i. Stem and leaf plot
ii. Bar diagram
iii. Box and whisker plot
iv. Line graph

Q.37. ***Inclusiveness, while developing case definitions for purposes of surveillance, would mean that the definition should be adequately*:**

i. Sensitive
ii. Specific
iii. Have high positive predictive value
iv. None of the above

Q.38. ***Who is called the founder of epidemiological surveillance*:**

i. Ramazzini
ii. John Graunt
iii. William Farr
iv. John Snow

Q.39. ***The very first step in investigation of an epidemic is*:**

i. Confirmation of existence of an epidemic
ii. Verification of diagnosis
iii. Develop epidemiological case sheet
iv. Formulation of hypothesis

Q.40. ***A nominal roll of the cases which have already been reported to the various health care establishments (like dispensaries, general practitioners or admitted to the hospitals) till the present moment would form*:**

i. Line list
ii. Epidemiological list
iii. Case summary
iv. Secondary data

Q.41. ***For purposes of terming a health-related event as an epidemic, the incidence rate computed is compared with the rate occurring in the same population, during the corresponding period of the past:***

i. 1 year
ii. 3 years
iii. 10 years
iv. No specific time frame is laid down

Q.42. ***All of the following categories are to be defined in developing valid case definitions of diseases, except:***

i. Suspect
ii. Fatal
iii. Probable
iv. Confirmed

Q.43. ***While developing an epidemiological case sheet in investigation of an epidemic, it would be prudent to go back by what time period from the onset of the first symptom, so as to get an idea of the agent to be incriminated:***

i. Maximum incubation period
ii. Minimum incubation period
iii. Latent period
iv. Range of incubation period

Q. 44. ***In case of large populations, while looking out for additional cases to complete the line list when investigating an epidemic, which type of sample should be ideally taken:***

i. Cluster sample
ii. Multistage sample
iii. Systematic random sample
iv. Stratified random sample

Q.45. ***An epidemic is described in all of the following ways/ parameters, except:***

i. According to time characteristics
ii. According to space characteristics
iii. According to person characteristics
iv. According to place characteristics

Q.46. ***Which test of significance is to be used while making comparisons using analytical techniques, between those who suffered, and those who did not suffer, though being a part of same source population, for testing the hypothesis in investigation of an epidemic:***

i. Paired t-test
ii. Unpaired t-test
iii. z-test
iv. Chi-square test

Q.47. ***All of the following are measures directed towards control and prevention of the source of infection, in an epidemic, once identified, except:***

i. Vector control measures
ii. Notification
iii. Isolation if required
iv. Detection and treatment of cases and carriers

Q.48. ***All of the following are measures directed towards protection of susceptible population, in an epidemic, once identified, except:***

i. Immunization
ii. Chemoprophylaxis
iii. Personal protective measures
iv. Quarantine

Q.49. ***For a study assessing the role of an exposure in leading to an outcome, what is the correct hierarchy as per strength of the design:***

i. Experimental > Cohort > Cross-sectional analytic and Case control > Ecological
ii. Ecological > Experimental > Cohort > Cross-sectional analytic and Case control
iii. Experimental > Cross-sectional analytic and Case control> Cohort > Ecological
iv. Cohort > Experimental > Cross-sectional analytic and Case control > Ecological

Q. 50. ***Which of the following should be examined to decide whether one should further read a particular article in detail:***

i. Title
ii. Abstract

iii. Material and method
iv. All of the above

Q.51. ***What are available methods for a researcher to control for potential confounding factors (PCFs) by taking action during design stage?***

i. Randomization
ii. Restriction
iii. Matching
iv. All of the above

Q.52. ***What are available methods for a researcher to control for PCFs during analysis?***

i. Standardization
ii. Stratified analysis
iii. Mathematical modeling
iv. All of the above

Q.53. ***The strength of association is seen by:***

i. Relative risk
ii. Odds ratio
iii. Both i and ii
iv. None of the above

Q.54. ***To see whether a diagnostic test really contributed to better patient management or favorably changed the disease outcome for which the test is designed, which of the following parameter is used:***

i. Validity
ii. Reliability
iii. Utility
iv. None of the above

Q.55. ***Randomization is an important step for:***

i. A study assessing the role of a risk factor/causal factors
ii. A study dealing with clinical course and prognostic factors
iii. A study on evaluation of a diagnostic test
iv. A study assessing the efficacy of a therapeutic or preventive procedure

Q.56. ***Which is false about institutional ethical committee?***

i. The chairperson should be an eminent person with a well-documented record in health research
ii. The chairperson should be from within the institution
iii. The secretary should be from within the institution
iv. It reviews and clears research proposals before they are actually launched

Q.57. ***Method to resolve the conflicts of interest in a research is:***

i. Scrutinizing research proposal carefully by the IEC
ii. Ensuring rigorous randomization
iii. By disclosing all possible conflicts in their published article
iv. All of the above

Q.58. ***Which of the following is not characteristic of qualitative research?***

i. Provides depth of understanding
ii. Study motivations/intentions/reasons
iii. Provide proof
iv. Study design is iterative

Q.59. ***Which of the following is characteristic of qualitative research?***

i. Predict causal relationships
ii. Describe relationship between variables
iii. Measure level of confidence
iv. Describe individual experiences

Q.60. ***Which of the following is not a method of data collection in qualitative research?***

i. Participant observation
ii. Interactive interviewing
iii. Written descriptions by participants
iv. None

Answer with explanation

Ans. 1. v. Epidemiology has been variously described by different authors ranging from Hippocrates to the present day. However, comprehensive definition of the science of epidemiology has been rendered by John M Last in 1988 as, "the study of the distribution and determinants of the health-related states or events in specified populations and the application of this study to the control of health problems".

Ans. 2. i. Incidence rate measures occurrence of new cases whereas prevalence rate is conglomerate of new as well as pre-existing cases, thus denoting the total burden of the disease.

Ans. 3. ii. Cohort study is a longitudinal study in which the number of new cases of a particular disease under study automatically gets counted as the study progresses.

Ans. 4. iii. The simplest tool available for rapid determination of prevalence is a cross-sectional study. It is basically an observational study and includes a single examination of a cross-section of the entire or representative sample of a population at a single point in time. The results can usually be extrapolated to the whole population. Cross-sectional studies are more useful for chronic diseases like hypertension, diabetes mellitus, etc. Such studies contribute neither towards establishing natural history of a disease nor its causal association.

Ans. 5. iv. To understand the above situation, the example of antiretroviral therapy (ART) in case of AIDS can be considered, wherein ART prolongs the life but does not cure AIDS, hence the prevalence of AIDS continues to increase.

Ans. 6. iv. Since case control studies proceed backward from effect to cause, they mainly indicate statistical association between exposure and occurrence of disease. Statistical association does not imply causation, however, strength of this association can be measured by odds ratio.

Ans. 7. ii. Relative risk (also known as risk ratio) is an estimate of disease risk associated with an exposure to a risk factor. Case control studies do not provide incidence rates from which relative risk can be calculated directly as these is no denominator or population available. Relative risk, therefore, can be determined exactly only from a cohort study.

Ans. 8. iii. The drop-out rate increases.

Ans. 9. ii. Avoid observer bias and sampling variation.

Ans. 10. i. Contagious disease is the one which is transmitted through contact, e.g. scabies, sexually transmitted diseases (STDs), trachoma, etc. Communicable disease is an illness due to a specific infectious agent or its toxic products capable of being directly or indirectly transmitted from man to man, animal to man, man to animal or animal to animal or from environment to man or animal. Infectious disease and communicable disease are both generic terms used interchangeably.

Ans. 11. iii. Subclinical cases are also referred to as 'missed' or 'abortive' cases, 'inapparent' or 'covert' cases. The disease agent may multiply in the host but does not manifest itself by signs and symptoms. These cases are equally important as sources of infection, hence maintain endemicity in an area by constantly shedding disease agent. On the other hand, some of cases harbor disease agent but do not shed the same in the community. The disease agent lies dormant within the host and may not be detectable in blood, tissues or other secretions. For such a situation, the term 'latent infection' is used.

Ans. 12. ii. Measles.

Ans. 13. iii. Japanese encephalitis.

Ans. 14. iv. Primary response depends on the dose of antigen, to the extent that with a small dose only IgM response may be elicited which is immediate. IgG response peaks in 7–10 days but needs about 50 times the dose of antigen. An important outcome of the primary response is development of 'immunological memory' based on B and T lymphocytes. The accelerated secondary response on a subsequent antigenic stimulus (booster) is the result of this immunological memory.

Ans. 15. iii. Response lasts for a shorter period.

Ans. 16. ii. The EPI was originally started by WHO in 1974 and was adopted by the Government of India in 1978. It included only BCG, DPT and typhoid for children under 5 years of age. It did not include measles vaccine and OPV was added in 1979. This program continued upto 1987. EPI was supplanted by Universal Immunization Program (UIP) in 1985. The Government of India subsequently set up the 'Technology mission on vaccination and immunization of vulnerable populations, specially children'. The UIP is current till now and is integral part of Reproductive and Child Health (RCH) Program since 1997. The immunization activities in India are largely supported by UNICEF.

Ans. 17. iv. 'Antisepsis' relates to destruction or inhibition of micro-organisms in living tissues, e.g. Savlon, Dettol, Chlorhexidine, etc. Deodorant is a substance which suppresses or neutralizes bad odors, e.g. lime, bleaching powder. 'Detergents' are surface cleaning agents and act by lowering the surface tension thereby breaking up the fat covering of dirt, e.g. soap. Disinfection is the killing of infectious agents outside the body by direct exposure to chemical or physical agents. The term is usually applied to inanimate objects or surfaces, e.g. phenol, sunlight, cresol, hypochlorite solution, etc. Chemical disinfectants in small doses or dilutions can also act as antiseptics.

Ans. 18. ii. Absolute alcohol is not effective against spores, hence cannot be termed as complete sterilizing agent.

Ans. 19. iv. None of the above.

Ans. 20. i. Highly sensitive test.

Ans. 21. i. Sensitivity.

That is, any person who has the disease being looked for should be identified as positive by the measurement process.

Ans. 22. i. Prevalence.

Prevalence is the proportion of persons "having" (i.e. found to be present with) the disease (or any other health-related condition of interest), out of the total subjects who were examined.

Ans. 23. ii. The disease should be vaccine preventable.

Ans. 24. iv. Longitudinal survey.

The essential feature which differentiates longitudinal survey with a cross-sectional one is that each subject is examined at least twice, to see the "change" that has occurred as regards the phenomena of interest over a period of time. These surveys measure the "incidence" and give a better insight into "cause and effect relationship".

Ans. 25. i. Repeated cross-sectional survey.

Hybrid surveys: These can often be used to obtain the advantages of both the cross-sectional as well as longitudinal surveys.

A very good example is "repeated cross-sectional surveys" which can give an approximate idea of the incidence. For example, if a cross-sectional survey in the year 1990 indicates that the prevalence of cervical cancer among women of reproductive age group is 1%, while another cross-sectional survey in the same population, in 2000, indicates the prevalence in the same population to be 2%, it may give a rough idea that the incidence of cervical cancer is (2–1) = 1% over 10 years.

Ans. 26. iv. Sampling frame.

A list of all the sampling units in the actual study population should be made which is known as the "sampling frame".

Ans. 27. iii. Universe.

Universe or reference population is very large, scattered and difficult to delimit, and hence representative sample cannot be directly drawn from it. For this reason, often specify a well-defined subset of the reference population from where the sample of subjects can be extracted.

Ans. 28. i. Provision of cash benefit.

Ans. 29. iii. Survey center method.

Ans. 30. iv. Urban elite.

Ans. 31. ii. To develop registries.

Ans. 32. iii. Completeness and accuracy.

Ans. 33. iv. Active surveillance.

In certain circumstances, data must be obtained by searching for cases (e.g. health workers go into the community, search for cases of fever and take their blood slide for malarial parasite), and also by periodically contacting those who may know of cases, as GPs, etc. For rare disease, or disease on way to eradication, or during outbreaks, active surveillance is necessary, so that cases which could have been otherwise missed, are promptly identified. Since, it is expensive, active surveillance is usually limited to specific diseases.

Ans. 34. iii. Academic interest.

Ans. 35. ii. Upper and lower control limits.

Analytic procedures usually are based on comparing the current incidence against the "Upper and Lower Control Limits" (UCL and LCL). [A quick method of calculating the UCL and LCL is UCL or LCL = R + 1.023 X A ; (Where R = Average of incidence rate per 1000 population for the corresponding period for the past 3 years and A is the average of "ranges" for the past 3 years. The resulting UCL and LCL will encompass 99% confidence interval)].

Ans. 36. iv. Line graph.

Ans. 37. i. Sensitive.

Ans. 38. iii. William Farr.

Ans. 39. ii. Verification of diagnosis.

Ans. 40. i. Line list.

A line list is like a nominal roll of the cases which have already been reported to the various health care establishments (like dispensaries, general practitioners or admitted to the hospitals) till now. Line listing of the cases is a major help in initial definition of the disease/syndrome that has occurred in epidemic form, in delineating the population at risk, and in preliminary definition of the transmission dynamics of the epidemic according to place and time.

Ans. 41. ii. 3 years.

Ans. 42. ii. Fatal.

Ans. 43. iv. Range of incubation period.

Ans. 44. iii. Systematic random sample.

Ans. 45. ii. According to space characteristics.

Ans. 46. iv. Chi-square test.

A chi-square (X^2) statistic is used to investigate whether distributions of categorical variables differ from one another. Basically categorical variable yield data in the categories and numerical variables yield data in numerical form.

Ans. 47. i. Vector control measures.

Ans. 48. iv. Quarantine.

Quarantine is compulsory isolation, typically to contain the spread of something considered dangerous, often but not always disease. The word comes from the Italian quarantena, meaning 40 day period. Quarantine can be applied to humans, but also to animals of various kinds.

Ans. 49. i. Experimental> Cohort> Cross-sectional analytic and Case control > Ecological.

Ans. 50. iv. All of the above.

Ans. 51. iv. All of the above.

Ans. 52. iv. All of the above.

Ans. 53. iii. Both (i) and (ii).

Ans. 54. iii. Utility.

For a study on evaluation of a diagnostic test, readers should examine the gold standard of diagnosis and whether all subjects were subjected to both tests. Check if study population had appropriate 'spectrum' of the target disease in form of mild, moderate, severe, atypical, and other closely related diagnoses. Also check the "settings" of study, referral filter, and reproducibility of the test under study. An important component is "utility" of the test, i.e. whether it really contributed to better patient management or favorably changed the disease outcome for which the test is designed.

Ans. 55. iv. A study assessing the efficacy of a therapeutic or preventive procedure.

Ans. 56. ii. The chairperson should be from within the institution.

Ans. 57. iv. All of the above.

Ans. 58. iii. Provide proof.

Qualitative research is often done to answer the question 'why' rather that 'what'. Quantitative research on the other hand involves techniques to quantify distribution and association of certain variables in a study population, mostly to provide proof rather than discovery.

Ans. 59. iv. Describe individual experiences.

Characteristics of qualitative research study.

a. Researcher focuses on the everyday life of people in natural settings.
b. The data have primacy; the theoretical framework is not predetermined but derives from the data.

c. Qualitative research is context bound—This means that the researcher has to be sensitive to the context of the research and immerse himself in the settings and the situation.
d. It focuses on the views of the people involved in the research and their perceptions, meanings and interpretations.
e. Data collection and analysis generally proceed together and interact with each other.
f. It uses open ended methods.
g. It involves respondents as active participants rather than subjects.

Ans. 60. iv. None.

3 Epidemiology of Communicable Diseases

Q.1. ***Presence of an infectious agent in an inanimate article or on skin surface, particularly hands, is called:***

i. Pollution
ii. Contamination
iii. Infection
iv. Infestation

Q.2. ***Which mode of transmission is followed in transmission of microfilaria through female culex mosquito?***

i. Cyclopropagative
ii. Propagative
iii. Cyclodevelopmental
iv. Vehicle-borne

Q.3. ***All of the followings are examples of direct modes of transmission except:***

i. Fomites
ii. Inoculation into skin or mucous membranes
iii. Droplet infection
iv. Vertical transmission

Q.4. ***Latent period + period of maximum communicability will give a crude estimate of the:***

i. Lead time
ii. Lag time
iii. Generation time
iv. Incubation period

Q.5. ***The level of immunity that is present in a population against an infectious agent is known as:***

i. Innate immunity
ii. Acquired immunity
iii. Selective immunity
iv. Herd immunity

Q.6. ***In calculation of secondary attack rate, exposure to which case is being taken into account:***

i. Primary case
ii. Index case
iii. Secondary case
iv. Subclinical case

Q.7. ***Case Fatality Ratio (CFR) is a reasonably good measure of:***

i. Pathogenicity
ii. Infectivity
iii. Virulence
iv. Infectiousness

Q.8. ***Epidemiologic chain of infection usually involves all of the following factors except:***

i. Disinfectants
ii. Infectious agent
iii. Human host
iv. Modes of transmission

Q.9. ***The presence and development of insect vectors on the body or linen, e.g. louse is known as:***

i. Infection
ii. Infestation
iii. Infectiousness
iv. Infectivity

Q.10. ***The time in which half of the infected subjects will develop clinical manifestations, following entry of the organism into the body, is known as:***

i. Lead time
ii. Median latent period
iii. Median incubation period
iv. Generation time

Q.11. ***That subset of endemic frequency, wherein exposure to infection generally occurs during early childhood so that by the time adulthood is achieved, the population becomes immune and a high level of herd immunity occurs, is known as:***

i. Hyperendemic
ii. Holoendemic

iii. Mesoendemic
iv. Hypoendemic

Q.12. ***Wassermann antibodies and bactericidal antibodies against gram-negative organisms (endotoxins) are almost exclusively found in:***

i. IgG
ii. IgM
iii. IgA
iv. IgE

Q.13. ***The objective of prevention and control measures in the prepathogenic phase is to achieve:***

i. Primary prevention
ii. Secondary prevention
iii. Tertiary prevention
iv. None of the above

Q.14. ***Broad categories of disinfecting agents are all except:***

i. Natural agents
ii. Physical agents
iii. Chemical agents
iv. Gaseous agents

Q.15. ***The temperature of the air in the oven should be maintained at:***

i. 160°C for at least one hour
ii. 170°C for at least one hour
iii. 180°C for at least one hour
iv. 190°C for at least one hour

Q.16. ***Steam introduced at pressure in excess of atmospheric pressure is known as:***

i. Current steam
ii. Unconfined steam
iii. Saturated steam
iv. Confined steam

Q.17. ***The underlying principle of "Syndromic Approach" to communicable disease surveillance is that the case definition is based on:***

i. A specific disease
ii. A group of diseases

iii. A syndrome
iv. None of the above

Q.18. ***Serum should be separated from blood prior to transportation if the time taken to reach the laboratory is:***

i. > 6 hours
ii. > 12 hours
iii. > 18 hours
iv. > 24 hours

Malaria

Q.19. ***Malignant tertian malaria is caused by:***

i. *Plasmodium vivax*
ii. *Plasmodium malariae*
iii. *Plasmodium falciparum*
iv. *Plasmodium ovale*

Q.20. ***The cyclopropagative life cycle of the plasmodium occurs in stages of:***

i. 2
ii. 3
iii. 4
iv. 5

Q.21. ***Most of the severe morbidity and mortality in malaria is caused by:***

i. *Plasmodium vivax*
ii. *Plasmodium malariae*
iii. *Plasmodium falciparum*
iv. *Plasmodium ovale*

Q.22. ***In order to infect a mosquito, the blood of a human carrier must contain at least how many gametocytes per mm^3:***

i. 10
ii. 12
iii. 14
iv. 16

Q.23. ***Main vector of malaria in Andaman and Nicobar Islands is:***

i. Anopheles dirus
ii. Anopheles sundaicus

iii. Anopheles maculatus
iv. Anopheles stephensi

Q.24. ***A hyperendemic area is defined as one in which:***

i. Spleen rate or parasite rate consistently over 10% in children between the ages of 2 and 9 years
ii. Spleen rate or parasite rate consistently over 30% in children between the ages of 2 and 9 years
iii. Spleen rate or parasite rate consistently over 50% in children between the ages of 2 and 9 years
iv. Spleen rate or parasite rate consistently over 75% in children between the ages of 2 and 9 years

Q.25. ***Rapid diagnostic test of malaria based on detection of antibodies against histidine-rich protein 2 is used for diagnosis of:***

i. *Plasmodium falciparum*
ii. *Plasmodium vivax*
iii. *Plasmodium ovale*
iv. All of the above

Q.26. ***Gold-standard in confirming the diagnosis of malaria is:***

i. Peripheral smear examination
ii. Immunochromatographic test
iii. Polymerase chain reaction
iv. Radioimmunoassay

Q.27. ***Drug of choice in severe and complicated malaria of Plasmodium falciparum:***

i. Artesunate
ii. Quinine
iii. Chloroquine
iv. None of the above

Q.28. ***In severe and complicated malaria recommended dose of Quinine is:***

i. 2.5 mg/kg body weight 8 hourly
ii. 5 mg/kg body weight 8 hourly
iii. 10 mg/kg body weight 8 hourly
iv. 15 mg/kg body weight 8 hourly

Lymphatic Filariasis

Q.29. ***Most prevalent parasitic worm in India:***

i. *Wuchereria bancrofti*
ii. *Brugia malayi*
iii. *Brugia timori*
iv. None of the above

Q.30. ***Brugia timori has only been found in parts of:***

i. South India
ii. Indonesia
iii. China
iv. Bangladesh

Q.31. ***The most important vector for lymphatic filariasis in India:***

i. Culex quinquefasciatus
ii. Culex tritaeniorhynchus
iii. Mansonia annulifera
iv. Mansonia uniformis

Q.32. ***Drug most widely used for treatment of lymphatic filariasis:***

i. Diethylcarbamazine (DEC)
ii. Ivermectin
iii. Albendazole
iv. None of the above

Leishmaniasis

Q.33. ***The disease is endemic in following three countries of the WHO South East Asia region except:***

i. Bangladesh
ii. India
iii. Nepal
iv. Sri Lanka

Q.34. ***The disease is reported in number of districts in India are:***

i. 51
ii. 52
iii. 53
iv. 54

Q.35. ***State which accounts for more than 90% of the cases in India:***

i. Uttar Pradesh

ii. Bihar
iii. Assam
iv. Madhya Pradesh

Q.36. *Leishmania donovani complex comprises of all except*:

i. *Leishmania infantum*
ii. *Leishmania chagasi*
iii. *Leishmania venezuelensis*
iv. *Leishmania donovani*

Q.37. *Cutaneous leishmaniasis is also known as all the following except*:

i. Oriental sore
ii. Aleppo evil
iii. Delhi boil
iv. Espundia

Dengue and Dengue Hemorrhagic Fever

Q.38. *Prior to 1970 the number of countries had experienced DHF epidemic are*:

i. 3
ii. 5
iii. 7
iv. 9

Q.39. *The city has reported the first major outbreak in India during 1963 is*:

i. Mumbai
ii. Kolkata
iii. Delhi
iv. Chennai

Q.40. *Dengue virus has how many serotypes*:

i. 2
ii. 4
iii. 6
iv. 8

Q.41. *IgM antibodies against dengue virus appear around how many days after onset of symptoms*:

i. 3
ii. 5

iii. 7
iv. 9

Japanese Encephalitis

Q.42. ***Japanese encephalitis virus is:***

i. Single–stranded RNA virus
ii. Double–stranded RNA virus
iii. Single–stranded DNA virus
iv. Double–stranded DNA virus

Q.43. ***In India principal vector for JE is:***

i. Culex quinquefasciatus
ii. Culex tritaeniorhynchus
iii. Aedes vittatus
iv. Aedes niveus

Q.44. ***Natural host for the virus are:***

i. Humans
ii. Cattle
iii. Pigs
iv. Monkeys

Q.45. ***Cell culture–derived vaccine is based on a specific strain of the JE virus which is:***

i. SA 14–14–1
ii. SA 15–15–1
iii. SA 14–14–2
iv. SA 15–15–2

Rickettsial Diseases

Q.46. ***Limited area of intensive transmission of rickettsiae called as:***

i. Typhus island
ii. Mite islands
iii. Rickettsiae island
iv. None of the above

Q.47. ***Agent for Indian Tick Typhus is:***

i. *Rickettsia typhi*
ii. *Rickettsia conorii*

iii. *Rickettsia akari*
iv. *Rickettsia prowazekii*

Q.48. ***Most commonly reported rickettsial infection in India is:***

i. Scrub typhus
ii. Indian tick typhus
iii. Epidemic typhus
iv. Rickettsial pox

Q.49. ***Epidemic typhus is transmitted by:***

i. Tick
ii. Mite
iii. Human louse
iv. Rat flea

Q.50. ***The infection is transmitted to man through the bite of infective mite in the form of:***

i. Larvae
ii. Pupa
iii. Male adult
iv. Female adult

Yellow Fever

Q.51. ***All the following are countries considered to be at high-risk for yellow fever except:***

i. Brazil
ii. Colombia
iii. Hong Kong
iv. Peru

Q.52. ***Principal urban vector of yellow fever is:***

i. *Aedes aegypti*
ii. *Aedes africanus*
iii. *Aedes simpsoni*
iv. *Aedes vittatus*

Q.53. ***The principal vector for forest transmission of yellow fever in South America is:***

i. *Aedes simpsoni*
ii. *Haemagogus spegazzinii*

iii. *Aedes vittatus*
iv. *Aedes niveus*

Q.54. *Strain of yellow fever virus used for vaccination*:

i. 16 D
ii. 17 D
iii. 18 D
iv. 19 D

Q.55. *The international yellow fever vaccination certificate becomes valid after how many days*:

i. 10
ii. 15
iii. 20
iv. 25

Plague

Q.56. *Yersinia pestis was first discovered in*:

i. 1893
ii. 1894
iii. 1895
iv. 1896

Q.57. *Number of species in the genus Yersinia considered important human pathogens*:

i. 1
ii. 3
iii. 5
iv. 7

Q.58. *Human flea responsible for human to human transmission of plague*:

i. *Pulex irritans*
ii. *Oropsylla montanus*
iii. *Nosopsyllus fasciatus*
iv. *Xenopsylla vexabilis*

Q.59. *Epizootic hosts are all except*:

i. Amplification hosts
ii. Maintenance hosts
iii. Highly susceptible
iv. Have high mortality

Q.60. ***The least common but most dangerous plague is:***

i. Septicemic plague
ii. Bubonic plague
iii. Pneumonic plague
iv. None of the above

Q.61. ***Drug of choice for treatment of plague:***

i. Tetracyclines
ii. Chloramphenicol
iii. Ciprofloxacin
iv. Streptomycin

Q.62. ***Antibiotics of choice for prophylaxis:***

i. Tetracyclines
ii. Rifampicin
iii. Ciprofloxacin
iv. Streptomycin

Anthrax

Q.63. ***All are properties of Bacillus anthracis except:***

i. Gram-positive
ii. Spore-forming
iii. Nonmotile
iv. Hemolytic

Q.64. ***All are anthrax toxins except:***

i. Edema factor (EF)
ii. Swelling factor (SF)
iii. Lethal factor (LF)
iv. Protective antigen

Q.65. ***Bacillus anthracis is known to have how many strains:***

i. 1 (EF)
ii. 2
iii. 3
iv. 4

Q.66. ***Antibiotic of choice in treatment of anthrax:***

i. Penicillin
ii. Ciprofloxacin

iii. Tetracyclines
iv. Chloramphenicol

Q.67. ***The most common clinical form of presentation of anthrax is:***

i. Pulmonary anthrax
ii. Gastrointestinal anthrax
iii. Cutaneous anthrax
iv. Anthrax meningitis

Tetanus

Q.68. ***In South East Asia, following country has eliminated maternal and neonatal tetanus:***

i. India
ii. Bangladesh
iii. Myanmar
iv. None of the above

Q.69. ***In neonatal tetanus, the average incubation period is about:***

i. 4 days
ii. 7 days
iii. 11 days
iv. 15 days

Q.70. ***This is the most common form of clinical presentation of tetanus:***

i. Localized tetanus
ii. Generalized tetanus
iii. Cephalic tetanus
iv. Neonatal tetanus

Q.71. ***The only condition which mimics tetanus closely is:***

i. Strychnine poisoning
ii. Botulism poisoning
iii. Rabies
iv. None of the above

Q.72. ***A 37-week pregnant woman attends the antenatal clinic for the first time. The correct advice regarding immunization is:***

i. Nil immunization being too late
ii. One dose of TT

iii. One dose of TT along with ATS
iv. One dose of TT followed by ATS for the newborn

Rabies

Q.73. ***Rabies is found in all parts of India except:***

i. Maharashtra
ii. Gujarat
iii. Andaman and Nicobar Islands
iv. Uttar Pradesh

Q.74. ***Rabies virus is:***

i. Bullet-shaped
ii. Diamond-shaped
iii. Cone-shaped
iv. Round-shaped

Q.75. ***Fluorescent antibody detection test in diagnosis of rabies is done in:***

i. Blood
ii. Urine
iii. Skin biopsy
iv. Saliva

Q.76. ***The dose for Human Rabies Immunoglobulin (HRIG) is:***

i. 10 IU/kg body weight
ii. 20 IU/kg body weight
iii. 30 IU/kg body weight
iv. 40 IU/kg body weight

Hepatitis

Q.77. ***Which of the following viruses is transmitted only by feco-oral route?***

i. Hepatitis A
ii. Hepatitis B
iii. Hepatitis C
iv. Hepatitis E

Q.78. ***Which of the following statements is not true regarding hepatitis A?***

i. Incubation period is 15–45 days

ii. Maximum infectivity is 2 weeks before to 1 week after the onset of icterus
iii. Chronic carriers are responsible for epidemics
iv. 0.5% sodium hypochlorite is an effective disinfectant for feces of a patient

Q.79. ***Most common cause of epidemic of infective hepatitis is:***

i. Hepatitis A virus (HAV)
ii. Hepatitis B virus (HBV)
iii. Hepatitis C virus (HCV)
iv. Hepatitis E virus (HEV)

Q.80. ***Mortality in pregnant women is higher in outbreaks of:***

i. Hepatitis A
ii. Hepatitis B
iii. Hepatitis C
iv. Hepatitis E

Leptospirosis

Q.81. ***Weil's disease was first described by Adolf Weil in:***

i. 1884
ii. 1885
iii. 1886
iv. 1887

Q.82. ***Drug used in chemoprophylaxis of leptospirosis:***

i. Ciprofloxacin
ii. Septran
iii. Doxycycline
iv. Rifampicin

Q.83. ***Inada and Ido identified the causal organism of leptospirosis in:***

i. America
ii. Japan
iii. S Korea
iv. China

Q.84. ***Humans are:***

i. Dead end host for leptospirosis
ii. Intermediate host for leptospirosis

iii. Amplifying host for leptospirosis
iv. None of the above

Brucellosis

Q.85. ***Brucellae are all except*:**

i. Motile
ii. Nonsporing
iii. Nontoxogenic
iv. Nonfermenting

Q.86. ***Animal reservoirs of Brucella suis is*:**

i. Buffalo
ii. Camels
iii. Feral swine
iv. Goats

Q.87. ***Brucellae causes abortion in*:**

i. Animals only
ii. Human beings only
iii. Both animals and human beings
iv. None of the above

Q.88. ***Drug of choice in treatment Brucella is*:**

i. Streptomycin
ii. Rifampicin
iii. Gentamicin
iv. Doxycycline

Measles

Q.89. ***The most common cause of death associated with measles is*:**

i. Measles encephalitis
ii. Pneumonia
iii. Subacute sclerozing panencephalitis
iv. Severe diarrhea

Q.90. ***Measles virus is*:**

i. Single-stranded RNA virus
ii. Double-stranded RNA virus
iii. Single-stranded DNA virus
iv. Double-stranded DNA virus

Q.91. ***Immunity lasts for _____ after natural infection:***

i. 5 years
ii. 10 years
iii. Lifelong
iv. None of the above

Q.92. ***A live attenuated vaccine against measles has been available since:***

i. 1964
ii. 1965
iii. 1966
iv. 1967

Q.93. ***The dose of human immunoglobulin for passive immunization against measles is:***

i. 0.25 ml/kg body weight
ii. 0.50 ml/kg body weight
iii. 0.75 ml/kg body weight
iv. 1.00 ml/kg body weight

Rubella

Q.94. ***The rubella virus is from __________ family:***

i. Herpesviridae
ii. Togaviridae
iii. Flaviviridae
iv. Paramyxoviridae

Q.95. ***Rubella virus has a diameter of:***

i. 50 nm
ii. 60 nm
iii. 70 nm
iv. 80 nm

Q.96. ***Rubella cases are infective from _____ days before to _____ days after onset of rash respectively:***

i. 2 and 4
ii. 8 and 10
iii. 10 and 15
iv. 20 and 15

Q.97. ***Average incubation period of rubella is:***

i. 16 days
ii. 18 days

iii. 20 days
iv. 22 days

Q.98. ***Rubella vaccine in India as MMR is given at:***

i. 6th month
ii. 9th month
iii. 15–18th month
iv. 20–24th month

Chickenpox and Herpes Zoster

Q.99. ***Chickenpox occurs in _________ forms in India:***

i. Endemic forms
ii. Epidemic forms
iii. Both endemic and epidemic
iv. None of the above

Q.100. ***The varicella zoster virus is a:***

i. Single-stranded RNA virus
ii. Double-stranded RNA virus
iii. Single-stranded DNA virus
iv. Double-stranded DNA virus

Q.101. ***Mortality rates in normal young children are estimated to be:***

i. Less than 1/100,000
ii. Less than 2/100,000
iii. Less than 3/100,000
iv. Less than 4/100,000

Q.102. ***The diagnosis of chickenpox is usually based on:***

i. Smear of vesicular fluid examination
ii. Serology
iii. Blood test
iv. History of exposure and clinical features

Q.103. ***Disseminated herpes zoster may occur in patients suffering from:***

i. Malignancies
ii. AIDS
iii. Immunocompromised states
iv. All of the above

Diphtheria

Q.104. ***The diphtheria bacillus was first described by:***

i. Klebs
ii. Loeffler
iii. Robert Koch
iv. None of the above

Q.105. ***The most important factor determining virulence of Corynebacterium diphtheriae is:***

i. Exotoxin
ii. Edotoxin
iii. O antigens
iv. K antigens

Q.106. ***This is the commonest site for respiratory diphtheria is:***

i. Anterior nasal
ii. Faucial infection
iii. Laryngeal or tracheobronchial infection
iv. None of the above

Q.107. ***This is the most severe type of respiratory infection:***

i. Anterior nasal
ii. Faucial infection
iii. Laryngeal or tracheobronchial infection
iv. None of the above

Q.108. ***All are characteristics of Corynebacterium diphtheriae except:***

i. Nonmotile
ii. Nonsporulating
iii. Encapsulated
iv. Gram-positive bacilli

Meningococcal Meningitis

Q.109. ***How many serogroups of Neisseria meningitides have been described?***

i. 13
ii. 14
iii. 15
iv. 16

Q.110. ***The predominant serogroups in Asia and Africa are:***

i. A and B
ii. B and C
iii. A and C
iv. B and 135

Q.111. ***The average incubation period is:***

i. 1–2 days
ii. 3–4 days
iii. 5–7 days
iv. 7–10 days

Q.112. ***Typical CSF abnormalities include all except:***

i. Increased pressure
ii. Decreased glucose concentration
iii. Predominantly neutrophils
iv. Decreased protein concentration

Q.113. ***Drug of choice for the treatment of meningococcal meningitis and septicemia is:***

i. Ampicillin
ii. Penicillin
iii. Chloramphenicol
iv. Cefotaxime

Tuberculosis

Q.114. ***Which disease is known as 'Captain of the Men of Death'?***

i. Tuberculosis
ii. AIDS
iii. Plague
iv. Cholera

Q.115. ***Pulmonary tuberculosis accounts for over ______ % of the total cases:***

i. 50%
ii. 60%
iii. 70%
iv. 80%

Q.116. ***The most common opportunistic infection in patients suffering from AIDS:***

i. Candidiasis
ii. Pulmonary tuberculosis

iii. Herpes
iv. Scabies

Q.117. ***The ________ region has the highest incidence rate per capita (363 per 1,00,000 population):***

i. Asian
ii. American
iii. Indian
iv. African

Q.118. ***_________ is the highest TB burden country in the world:***

i. Nigeria
ii. South Africa
iii. India
iv. Bangladesh

Q.119. ***It is estimated that a cough can generate _____.***

i. 1000 droplet nuclei
ii. 2000 droplet nuclei
iii. 3000 droplet nuclei
iv. 4000 droplet nuclei

Q.120. ***Under RNTCP in reporting of sputum smears, 1–10 AFB per oil immersion field is graded as:***

i. 1+
ii. 2+
iii. 3+
iv. 4+

Q.121. ***Category III continuation phase comprises of:***

i. 4 H3 R3
ii. 5 H3 R3 E3
iii. 1 H3 R3 Z3 E3
iv. None of the above

Q.122. ***All new TB cases known to be HIV positive are treated with:***

i. Category I regimen
ii. Category II regimen
iii. Category III regimen
iv. None of the above

Q.123. ***Multidrug resistant (MDR) tuberculosis treatment involves all drugs except:***

i. Kanamycin
ii. Pyrazinamide

iii. Rifampicin
iv. Ethambutol

Avian Influenza

Q.124. ***The first documented infection of humans with an avian influenza virus occurred in:***

i. Vietnam
ii. China
iii. Hong Kong
iv. Bangladesh

Q.125. ***Spanish influenza pandemic occurred in the year:***

i. 1918
ii. 1957
iii. 1968
iv. 1970

Q.126. ***The optimal specimen for influenza A virus detection is:***

i. Blood
ii. Urine
iii. Stool
iv. Nasopharyngeal aspirate

Q.127. ***Recommended drug for chemoprophylaxis against H5N1 influenza is:***

i. Zanamivir
ii. Oseltamivir
iii. Amantadine
iv. Rimantadine

Q.128. ***Nonmedical interventions for defence against influenza pandemic are all except:***

i. Health education
ii. Stringent sanitary measures
iii. Vaccination
iv. Appropriate biosecurity practices

Severe Acute Respiratory Syndrome (SARS)

Q.129. ***Country which has reported maximum number of cases of SARS:***

i. Canada

ii. Singapore
iii. Hong Kong
iv. China

Q.130. ***All of the following states in India reported probable cases of SARS in 2003 except:***

i. West Bengal
ii. Karnataka
iii. Andhra Pradesh
iv. Gujarat

Q.131. ***SARS corona virus is:***

i. Enveloped RNA virus
ii. Nonenveloped RNA virus
iii. Enveloped DNA virus
iv. Nonenveloped DNA virus

Q.132. ***SARS virus can survive after drying on plastic surfaces for upto:***

i. 24 hours
ii. 48 hours
iii. 72 hours
iv. 96 hours

Q.133. ***Immunofluorescence Assays (IFA) detect antibodies in serum of SARS patients_____ days after the onset of illness:***

i. 5
ii. 10
iii. 15
iv. 20

Helminthiasis

Q.134. ***In the classification of communities based on prevalence and intensity of infection of soil-transmitted helminthic infections, a high-transmission community is one wherein:***

i. Prevalence greater than 50%, heavy infection less than 10%
ii. Prevalence less than 50%, heavy infection less than 10%
iii. Prevalence greater than 10%, heavy infection less than 50%

iv. Prevalence greater than 50%, heavy infection more than 10%

Q.135. ***All of the following are types of soil-transmitted helminthes based on the life cycle, except:***

i. Direct
ii. Indirect
iii. Penetration of the skin
iv. Modified direct

Q.136. ***All of the following are examples of food borne helminthes examples except:***

i. *Wuchereria bancrofti*
ii. *Clonorchis sinensis*
iii. *Fasciola hepatica*
iv. *Fasciola buski*

Q.137. ***Retrograde infection is a significant mode of transmission of:***

i. Ascariasis (roundworm)
ii. Paragonimus (lung fluke)
iii. Enterobius (threadworm)
iv. Ankylostoma (hookworm)

Q.138. ***For whipworm infection to be termed as heavy infection, the number of eggs per gram of feces is more than or equal to:***

i. 10000
ii. 20000
iii. 30000
iv. 40000

Q.139. ***In areas where ascariasis is endemic and maximum prevalence is found in preschool and primary school age children, intensity of infection in adults low, transmission household or family type, the pattern is known as:***

i. Mild prevalence
ii. Moderate prevalence
iii. Intense prevalence
iv. High prevalence

Q.140. ***A safe and effective drug in the management of ascariasis in a pregnant woman is:***

i. Praziquantel
ii. Mebendazole
iii. Albendazole
iv. Pyrantel pamoate

Q.141. ***Diphyllobothrium latum (fish tapeworm) in its life cycle, passes through:***

i. 1 definitive host and 2 intermediate hosts
ii. 2 definitive hosts and 1 intermediate host
iii. 1 definitive host and 1 intermediate host
iv. 2 definitive hosts and 2 intermediate hosts

Q.142. ***Drug of choice in cases of cysticercosis is:***

i. Albendazole
ii. Mebendazole
iii. Praziquantel
iv. pyrantel pamoate

Q.143. ***Consumption of raw or incompletely cooked crabs, crayfish and shrimps harboring metacercariae, leads to infection with:***

i. Liver fluke
ii. Lung fluke
iii. Blood fluke
iv. Intestinal fluke

Q.144. ***Reservoir of infection in man, in cases of intestinal fluke (Fasciola hepatica) is:***

i. Pig
ii. Cow
iii. Snail
iv. Dog

Q.145. ***Encysted larvae in muscles of pork, when ingested, is the infective form in cases of infection with:***

i. Fasciola hepatica (liver flukes)
ii. Trichinella spiralis (trichina worm)
iii. Ascaris lumbricoides (roundworm)
iv. Paragonimus westermani (lung flukes)

Q.146. ***What amount of iron is approximately lost in cases of chronic hookworm infection, leading to iron deficiency anemia:***

i. 10 mg of iron/10,000 ova/gm of feces
ii. 0.1 mg of iron/10,000 ova/gm of feces
iii. 5 mg of iron/10,000 ova/gm of feces
iv. 1 mg of iron/10,000 ova/gm of feces

Amebiasis and Giardiasis

Q.147. ***In India, the prevalence of amebiasis is:***

i. 5%
ii. 10%
iii. 15%
iv. 20%

Q.148. ***The form of E. histolytica usually infective to man is:***

i. Trophozoite
ii. Merozoite
iii. Egg
iv. Cyst

Q.149. ***Reservoir of infection of E. histolytica is:***

i. Housefly
ii. Man
iii. Soil
iv. Dog

Q.150. ***E. histolytica trophozoite causes ulceration commonly in:***

i. Rectum
ii. Duodenum
iii. Transverse and descending colon
iv. Cecum and ascending colon

Q.151. ***All are true of epidemiology of amebiasis except:***

i. No sex difference
ii. Does not affect children
iii. More among low socio-economic status
iv. Incubation period is 2–4 weeks

Q.152. ***Severe infection of E. histolytica occurs in all except:***

i. Very young children
ii. Pregnant women

iii. Malnourished individuals
iv. Patients with AIDS

Q.153. ***Drug of choice for amebic liver abscess is:***

i. Metronidazole
ii. Tinidazole
iii. Diloxanide furoate
iv. Iodoquinol

Q.154. ***Worldwide prevalence of amebiasis is:***

i. 5%
ii. 10%
iii. 15%
iv. 20%

Q.155. ***In outbreak circumstances the number of consecutive negative stool samples required for food handlers to return back to work is/are:***

i. 1
ii. 2
iii. 3
iv. 4

Q.156. ***The trophozoite of Giardia lamblia inhabits:***

i. Cecum
ii. Rectum
iii. Ascending and transverse colon
iv. Duodenum and upper jejunum

Q.157. ***What percentage of Traveller's diarrhea is due to Giardia infections:***

i. 8%
ii. 12%
iii. 16%
iv. 20%

Sexually Transmitted Infections (STI)

Q.158. ***Main aims of STD control are:***

i. To interrupt the transmission of sexually acquired infections
ii. To prevent the development of diseases, complications and sequelae

iii. To reduce the risk of HIV infection
iv. All

Q.159. ***Vulnerable groups for STIs are all except:***

i. Commercial sex workers
ii. Men who have sex with men
iii. Couples in monogamous relationship
iv. Substance users, prisoners and young people

Q.160. ***Health education for STIs should include educational messages viz:***

i. Avoid sex with many different partners
ii. Description of treatment for different syndromes
iii. Description of recognizable signs and symptoms
iv. Advice on assessing one's personal risk of having acquired an STD

Q.161. ***The usual methods of early case detection is/are:***

i. Screening
ii. Contact tracing
iii. Cluster testing
iv. All

Q.162. ***Objective of case management of patients with STIs is/ are:***

i. To make a correct diagnosis
ii. To provide costly treatment
iii. To reduce/prevent future risk–taking behavior
iv. To advise on treatment compliance

Q163. ***Presence of vaginal discharge in syndromic management could be presentation of:***

i. Chlamydia
ii. Gonorrhea
iii. Bacterial vaginosis infection
iv. All

Q.164. ***All of the following are STIs except:***

i. *Ureaplasma urealyticum*
ii. Shigella
iii. *Candida albicans*
iv. Staphylococcus

Acquired Immunodeficiency Syndrome (AIDS)

Q.165. ***The risk of contracting HIV infection from transfusion of a unit of infected blood is estimated to be ____________ from infected mother to fetus:***

i. 15–30%
ii. 30–60%
iii. 10–15%
iv. 5–15%

Q.166. ***In adults for surveillance of AIDS major signs are all except:***

i. Weight loss > 10% of body weight
ii. Chronic diarrhea for more than 1 month
iii. Prolonged fever for more than 1 month
iv. Disseminated TB

Q.167. ***For children major signs for AIDS surveillance are all except:***

i. Weight loss or abnormally slow growth
ii. Chronic diarrhea for more than 1 month
iii. Prolonged fever for more than 1 month
iv. Persistent cough for more than 1 month

Q.168. ***Absolute CD4 count in HIV is used as:***

i. Screening test
ii. Confirmatory test
iii. Prognostic marker
iv. Diagnostic marker

Q.169. ***HIV can be transmitted from person to person through all methods except:***

i. Sexual contact
ii. Social contact
iii. Vertical transmission
iv. Blood transfusion

Q.170. ***Cytomegalovirus disease occurs when CD4 counts fall below:***

i. 200/cu mm
ii. 50/cu mm
iii. 500/cu mm
iv. 1000/cu mm

Q.171. ***Efavirenz belongs to:***

i. NRTI
ii. NNRTI
iii. PI
iv. Fusion inhibitors

Q.172. ***Postexposure prophylaxis should be started:***

i. Preferably within 1–2 hours
ii. Between 24–48 hours
iii. After 48 hours
iv. After 72 hours

Q.173. ***Currently, new infection rates and deaths due to HIV/AIDS are estimated from:***

i. HIV prevalence
ii. Average time between HIV infection and death in the absence of treatment
iii. Survival rates of people receiving treatment
iv. All

Q.174. ***Patients with a CD4+ count below 50 cells/mm^3 are at risk of developing disseminated***

i. *Mycobacterium avium* infection
ii. Cytomegalovirus disease
iii. PML
iv. All

Q.175. ***Obstetric practices will reduce the risk of mother to child transmission except:***

i. Avoidance of early rupture of membranes
ii. Conduct routine episiotomies
iii. Using nontraumatizing suction cups on vacuum extractors where possible
iv. Avoid fetal scalp puncture

Q.176. ***Who should be offered the HIV test:***

i. Persons with high-risk behavior
ii. Persons who request testing, regardless of risk
iii. Persons with certain medical conditions
iv. All

Leprosy (Hansen's Disease)

Q.177. ***Leprosy is also known as:***

i. Hansen's disease
ii. Koch's disease
iii. Crippling disease
iv. Weil's disease

Q.178. ***Contact surveillance of households in lepromatous case is recommended for the period of ________ years:***

i. 10
ii. 5
iii. 15
iv. 7

Q.179. ***Contact surveillance of households in nonlepromatous case is recommended for the period of ________ years:***

i. 10
ii. 5
iii. 15
iv. 7

Q.180. ***According to WHO, clinical classification multibacillary leprosy have:***

i. 5 or more lesions
ii. 6 or more lesions
iii. 5 lesions
iv. All of the above

Q.181. ***Lepromin test is read at ________ and ________:***

i. 24 hours and 21 days
ii. 48 hours and 21days
iii. 24 hours and 7 days
iv. 48 hours and 7 days

Q.182. ***Duration of paucibacillary leprosy treatment is:***

i. 6 months
ii. 9 months
iii. 12 months
iv. 18 months

Q.183. ***Classification into pauci and multibacillary leprosy is based on __________ features:***

i. Clinical
ii. Histological
iii. Bacteriological
iv. Immunological

Q.184. ***According to Indian classification, leprosy is classified into __________ types:***

i. 5
ii. 4
iii. 3
iv. 2

Answer with explanation

Ans. 1. ii. Contamination.

Refers to an infectious agent being present in inanimate articles like food, water, linen, patient care items or routine usage items like cutlery, toys, etc. often, the term is also used to denote presence of infectious agent on skin surface, particularly on hands.

Ans. 2. iii. Cyclodevelopmental.

When the agent undergoes developmental changes in the body of the vector but no multiplication takes place, it is known as "developmental" or "cyclodevelopmental" method.

Ans. 3. i. Fomites.

Defined as inanimate objects of general use by the infected person (e.g. utensils, linen, fountain pens, toothbrushes, etc.). The infectious agent may remain on the surface of such fomites and may be transmitted to the susceptible host usually when such objects are put into the mouth or come in contact with conjunctiva and helps in the indirect mode of transmission.

Ans. 4. iii. Generation time.

The generation time is the duration between the entry of infectious agent into the body to the peak infectivity of the host. As a crude calculation, generation time (G) is equal to (latent period + period of maximum communicability).

Ans. 5. iv. Herd immunity.

Herd immunity refers to the level of immunity that is present in a population against an infectious agent. It is, thus, concerned with the protection of a "population" from infection, the protection being brought about by the presence of immune individuals. It may be defined as "the resistance of a group to attack by a disease to which a large proportion of the members are immune, thus decreasing the probability that a person having the infectious agent will transmit it to another susceptible person in the same population".

Ans. 6. ii. Index case.
Secondary attack rate (SAR) is usually measured by conducting studies in closed communities or families wherein the first case which brings in the infection is called the index case.

Ans. 7. iii. Virulence.
It is the ability of the agent to produce severe disease.

Ans. 8. i. Disinfectants.

Ans. 9. ii. Infestation.

Ans. 10. iii. Median incubation period.
It is the time in which half of the infected subjects will develop clinical manifestations, following entry of the organism into the body.

Ans. 11. ii. Holo-endemic.

Ans. 12. ii. IgM.
Wassermann antibodies and bactericidal antibodies against gram-negative organisms (endotoxins) are almost exclusively found in IgM. It accounts for 5–10 percent of serum antibodies. It cannot pass through placenta. Normal adult serum level is 20–130 mg/100 ml.

Ans. 13. i. Primary prevention.

Ans. 14. iv. Gaseous agents.

Ans. 15. i. 160°C for at least one hour.

Ans. 16. iv. Confined steam.
Steam introduced at atmospheric pressure is known as 'current' or 'unconfined' steam: and at pressure in excess of that is called 'pressure' or 'confined steam'.

Ans. 17. iii. A syndrome.
The underlying principle of the "*syndromic approach*" to communicable disease surveillance and field investigation of an outbreak is that the

case definition is based on a syndrome and not on a specific disease, e.g. acute diarrheal syndrome.

Ans. 18. iv. 24 hours.

Ans. 19. iii. *Plasmodium falciparum.*

Ans. 20. i. 2.

The cyclopropagative life cycle of the Plasmodium occurs in two stages. The sexual stage starts with the 'gametogony' in the human host and progresses through 'sporogony' in the mosquito. The asexual stage starts with injection of sporozoites by the infective mosquito into the human host and progresses through three phases of 'schizogony'.

Ans. 21. iii. *Plasmodium falciparum.*

Ans. 22. ii. 12

For human plasmodia the only reservoir is a malaria case. In some parts of Africa, Chimpanzees may act as reservoir of *Plasmodium malariae.* The source of infection is a malaria case with adequate number of mature viable gametocytes circulating in the blood. It has been estimated that in order to infect a mosquito, the blood of a human carrier must contain at least 12 gametocytes per mm^3 and the number of female gametocytes must be more than the male gametocytes.

Ans. 23. ii. Anopheles sundaicus.

Places like Andaman and Nicobar Islands the main vector is Anopheles sundaicus which prefers to breed in brackish waters and fly upto 8 or 10 km.

Ans. 24. iii. Spleen rate or parasite rate consistently over 50% in children between the ages of 2 and 9 years.

Ans. 25. i. *Plasmodium falciparum.*

Ans. 26. i. Peripheral smear examination.

Microscopic examination of thick and thin peripheral blood smears stained with Romanowsky dye.

Ans. 27. ii. Quinine.

Ans. 28. iii. 10 mg/kg body weight 8 hourly.

Ans. 29. i. *Wuchereria bancrofti.*

Ans. 30. ii. Indonesia.

Ans. 31. i. Culex quinquefasciatus.

Ans. 32. i. Diethylcarbamazine (DEC).
Diethylcarbamazine (DEC) is the drug used most widely for treatment of lymphatic filariasis in 9–12 mg/kg orally in 3 divided doses. Other drugs used are Albendazole and Ivermectin. The use of single doses of two drugs administered together (Albendazole with DEC or Ivermectin) is 99% effective in removing microfilariae from the blood.

Ans. 33. iv. Sri Lanka.

Ans. 34. ii. 52.
India is one of the world's largest foci of visceral leishmaniasis, accounting for 50% of the total burden of this disease. Leishmaniasis is endemic in eastern states of India. A total of 52 districts in the country are considered endemic for the disease. An estimated 165.4 million population is at risk of kala- azar in 4 states. In India, about 1,00,000 cases of visceral leishmaniasis are estimated to occur annually.

Ans. 35. ii. Bihar.

Ans. 36. iii. Leishmania venezuelensis.
The human pathogens include the Leishmania donovani complex with 3 species (Leishmania donovani, Leishmania infantum and Leishmania chagasi). The Leishmania mexicana complex has 3 main species which are Leishmania mexicana, Leishmania amazonensis and Leishmania venezuelensis.

Ans. 37. iv. Espundia.
Mucosal leishmaniasis or Espundia where people infected, develops mucosal lesions in the nose,

mouth, pharynx, or larynx months to years after resolution of the primary skin lesion. The condition is known as Espundia in Latin America. Mucosal leishmaniasis often begins with nasal stuffiness and inflammation. Ulceration of the nasal mucosa and septum follows.

Ans. 38. iv. 9.

Ans. 39. ii. Kolkata.

Ans. 40. ii. 4.

DF/DHF is caused by dengue virus which belongs to genus Flavivirus family Flaviviridae and includes serotypes 1, 2, 3 and 4 (Den-1, Den-2, Den-3 and Den-4). The dengue virus is composed of single - stranded RNA. Each serotype provides specific lifetime immunity and short-term cross-immunity. All serotypes can cause severe and fatal disease. There are genetic variations within the serotypes. Some genetic variants within each serotype appear to be more virulent or have greater epidemic potential. When a person has had classic dengue, a second infection later by another serotype increases the likelihood of suffering from DHF as explained by the immune enhancement mechanism (1, 2, 4). Infection with one serotype provides life-long homologous immunity but does not provide protection against other serotypes, and instead may exacerbate subsequent infection (4, 6, 7).

Ans. 41. ii. 5.

Laboratory tests essential for confirmatory diagnosis of dengue infection include isolation of the virus, demonstration of a rising titer of specific serum dengue antibodies, and demonstration of a specific viral antigen or RNA in the tissue or serum. Serological diagnosis is based on detection of IgM antibodies. IgM antibodies against dengue virus appear around 5 days after onset of symptoms and are detectable for 1–3 months after the illness. The tests employed are IgM capture ELISA test and rapid IgM strip test. IgM capture ELISA test kit is available from NIV Pune and commercial sources and rapid IgM strip test kit is available commercially.

Ans. 42. i. Single-stranded RNA virus.

Ans. 43. ii. Culex tritaeniorhynchus.

In India and many endemic areas in Asia, Culex tritaeniorhynchus is the principal vector. This species feeds outdoors beginning at dusk and during evening hours until dawn. It breeds in water pools, marshes, flooded rice fields, and small stable collections of water around cultivated fields.

Ans. 44. iii. Pigs.

Pigs and aquatic birds (mainly herons and egrets of the Ardeidae family) are the natural hosts for the virus. Pigs are considered amplifying hosts since they allow manifold virus multiplication without suffering from disease and maintain prolonged viremia. Viremic adult pigs remain asymptomatic, but pregnant sows may abort or deliver stillbirths.

Ans. 45. iii. SA 14–14–2.

A live attenuated vaccine widely used in China is the cell culture-derived vaccine based on the SA 14–14 –2 strain of the JE virus. The World Health Organization recommends that JE immunization should be integrated into the EPI programs in all areas where JE constitutes a public health problem.

Ans. 46. i. Typhus Island.

The vector mite is now known to be present in diverse ecological niches such as equatorial rain forests, semi-deserts and Alpine subarctic terrains in the Himalayan regions. Endemic foci are usually associated with specific habitats such as abandoned plantations, gardens or rice fields, overgrown forest clearings, shrubby fringes of fields and forests, river banks and grassy fields. These ecological patches which attract the natural host of mite vectors are called “mite islands. Within the mite islands there may be a limited area of intensive transmission of rickettsia called "Typhus Island".

Ans. 47. ii. Rickettsia conorii.

Ans. 48. i. Scrub typhus.

Ans. 49. iii. Human louse.

The disease caused by Rickettsia mainly transmitted by the human louse *Pediculus humanus corporis*. The infection is transmitted by the entry of the infectious feces, the gut contents, or the body fluid of the louse through abrasion on the skin which may result from simultaneous scratching.

Ans. 50. i. Larvae.

The filariform larvae gain entrance to the human body by piercing the skin. There it enters the lymphatics and reaches pulmonary alveoli through lymphovascular system, right heart and pulmonary capillaries. They then migrate upwards the respiratory system and get ultimately swallowed. During its entry to esophagus, third moulting takes place and a terminal buccal capsule is formed. The growing larvae settle down in small intestine and undergo a fourth moulting to develop into adolescent worms. In 3–4 weeks time they become sexually mature and following fertilization, the female starts laying eggs. The whole cycle is completed in about 6 weeks.

Ans. 51. iii. Hong Kong.

Ans. 52. i. Aedes aegypti.

In India, Aedes aegypti is widespread and the people possess no immunity against yellow fever. Yellow fever has not so far entered India due to the stringent regulations and their rigid enforcement. It is, however, interesting to note that yellow fever never entered India even before these regulations were introduced. May be, this was due to the slow mode of voyage from the African coast to India.

Ans. 53. ii. Haemagogus spegazzinii.

Ans. 54. ii. 17 D.

This is the approved vaccine for international travel. It is a live, attenuated chick embryo grown 17D-strain freeze-dried vaccine. For storage at WHO approved centers, the vaccine can be kept for 3 months at +4°C. If the storage is for a longer duration, a temperature of –25°C is to be maintained. After reconstitution, it should be used within half an hour.

Ans. 55. i. 10.

More than 95% of vaccinated people develop neutralizing antibodies within 10–14 days of immunization. The International Health Regulations stipulate that the vaccination certificate for yellow fever is valid 10 days after administration of 17D vaccine, corresponding to the time at which the majority of vaccinees are demonstrably immune. Immunity following 17D vaccination is remarkably durable and may be lifelong.

Ans. 56. ii. 1894.

Ans. 57. ii. 3.

Ans. 58. i. Pulex irritans.

Pulex irritans, the human flea may be responsible for human to human transmission of plague.

Ans. 59. ii. Maintenance hosts.

More than 200 mammalian species have been known to be naturally infected with *Yersinia pestis*. However, plague is primarily a disease of rodents. The infection is maintained in natural foci of the disease in wild rodent colonies through transmission between rodents. The animal hosts of plague are classified as enzootic (maintenance) hosts and epizootic (amplification) hosts. Enzootic hosts are characterized by relatively mild illness, and low mortality rates. Voles and mice have been suggested as maintenance hosts. Epizootic rodents are associated with susceptibility and high mortality. Highly susceptible or epizootic plague hosts include various species of mice, rats, voles, gerbils, ground squirrels and marmots. Rats have historically been a primary carrier of plague.

Ans. 60. iii. Pneumonic plague.
Pneumonic plague is the least common but most dangerous and fatal form of the disease. It can develop as a secondary complication of septicemia plague or result from inhalation of infectious droplets.

Ans. 61. iv. Streptomycin.
Streptomycin is the drug of choice. The dose of streptomycin is 30 mg/kg/day (not more than of 2 gm/day) in divided doses given intramuscularly. Streptomycin must be given for a full course of 10 days or until 3 days after the temperature has returned to normal.

Ans. 62. i. Tetracyclines.
Tetracyclines are effective in the primary treatment of patients with uncomplicated plague. An oral loading dose of 15 mg/kg tetracycline (not to exceed 1 gm total) should be followed by 25–50 mg/kg/day (upto a total of 2 gm/day) for 10 days. Tetracyclines may also be used adjunctively with other antibiotics. Fluoroquinolones, such as ciprofloxacin are also effective.

Ans. 63. iv. Hemolytic.

Ans. 64. ii. Swelling factor (SF).
The virulence of the organism depends on the bacterial capsule and the toxin complex. The capsule is a poly-D-glutamic acid that protects it against lysis and phagocytosis. There are three anthrax toxins: The Edema Factor (EF), the Lethal Factor (LF) and a protective antigen.

Ans. 65. i. 1 Edema factor (EF).

Ans. 66. i. Penicillin.
Bacillus anthracis is highly sensitive to penicillin which is the antibiotic of choice. The pathogen is also sensitive to several other antibiotics including chloramphenicol, tetracycline, fluoroquinolones and erythromycin. In most cases

particularly inhalational and gastrointestinal anthrax, antibiotics must initially be administered intravenously. But according to CDC protocols, it is recommend Ciprofloxacin 400 mg BD or Doxycycline 100 mg BD for a total of 60 days. The dose of Ciprofloxacin for children is 10–15 mg/kg BD for 60 days. The treatment remains the same for pregnant women and immune compromised individuals.

Ans. 67. iii. Cutaneous anthrax.
This is the most common form of presentation accounting for over 95% of all cases. The incubation period can be as short as 9 hours to as long as 2 weeks, but usually ranges from 2–6 days. Over a period of approximately 10 days the cutaneous lesion which occurs at the site of entry of the spores, goes through the stages of a papule, ring of vesicles, ulceration and formation of a typical black eschar. The cutaneous lesion is nonpurulent and is typically painless. After 10 days the eschar begins to resolve. The resolution of the eschar occurs over 6 weeks and is not hastened by treatment. Cutaneous anthrax is self-limiting and in over 90% of cases resolution of the eschar takes place without complications.

Ans. 68. iv. None of the above.

Ans. 69. ii. 7 days.

Ans. 70. ii. Generalized tetanus.
Tetanus is the only noncommunicable disease that is vaccine preventable. It is an infectious disease caused by infection with *Clostridium tetani.* Under favorable anerobic conditions, the pathogen produces tetanospasmin, which is a potent neurotoxin. This toxin blocks inhibitory neurotransmitters in the central nervous system and causes the muscular stiffness and spasms typical of generalized tetanus.

Ans. 71. i. Strychnine poisoning.
A bedside diagnostic test called the 'spatula test' with very high specificity and sensitivity has been

proposed from India. Isolation of *Clostridium tetani* from can neither confirm nor exclude the diagnosis. The pathogen is often isolated from wounds among patients who do not have the disease and even carefully performed anerobic cultures are negative even from contaminated wounds. The only condition which mimics tetanus closely is strychnine poisoning. Serology also has little value as antibody levels even in the protective range do not rule out disease.

Ans. 72. iv. One dose of TT followed by ATS for the newborn. In a developing country like India due to poor antenatal coverage, it is not uncommon for pregnant women to present for the first time late in third trimester. As a golden rule, TT must be offered to the pregnant woman. However, the newborn still incurs the risk of neonatal tetanus, hence should be protected by injection of ATS 750 IU within 6 hours of birth.

Ans. 73. iii. Andaman and Nicobar Islands.

Ans. 74. i. Bullet-shaped.
The rabies viruses belong to the genus *Lyssavirus* of the *Rhabdoviridae* family. Currently, this genus comprises 7 genotypes, type 1 of which represents the classic rabies virus. This RNA virus is bullet-shaped round at one end and flat at the other measuring 100–300 nm in length and 75 nm in diameter. The virus is covered with a lipid envelope having spike like projections.

Ans. 75. iii. Skin biopsy.
Fluorescent antibody detection in skin biopsy (from neck) can be done for confirmation of diagnosis. Postmortem tests include demonstration of 'Negri bodies' and isolation of virus. It is important to distinguish rabies from treatable conditions to ensure protection of health care workers, prevent rabies hysteria/psychosis. It is also essential to distinguish rabies from postvaccinial encephalomyelitis caused by the nerve tissue vaccine.

Ans. 76. ii. 20 IU/kg body weight.
Rabies immunoglobulin of both equine (ERIG) and human (HRIG) is available. RIG should be administered in all category III exposures and in category II exposures involving immune deficient individuals. Given its relatively slow clearance, Human Rabies Immunoglobulin (HRIG) is the preferred product, particularly in cases of multiple severe exposures. Where HRIG is not available or affordable, purified Equine Immunoglobulin (ERIG) is used. Most of the new ERIG preparations are potent, highly purified, safe and considerably less expensive than HRIG. The dose for HRIG is 20 IU/kg body weight, and for ERIG is 40 IU/kg body weight. As much of the recommended dose of passive immunization products as is anatomically feasible should be infiltrated into and around the wounds. The remainder should be administered by deep intramuscular injection at an injection site distant from the vaccine injection site. In case of multiple wounds, the RIG should be diluted with normal saline to make sufficient volume to ensure infiltration at all wound sites. RIG for passive immunization should not be injected later than 7 days after the initiation of postexposure vaccination.

Ans. 77. iv. Hepatitis E.
Although hepatitis A is predominantly transmitted by feco-oral route, it is also known to be transmitted by parenteral and sexual route albeit uncommonly.

Ans. 78. iii. Chronic carriers are responsible for epidemics.

Ans. 79. iv. Hepatitis E virus (HEV).

Ans. 80. iv. Hepatitis E.
HEV is also known to have a propensity to induce fulminant hepatic failure with mortality range from 0.5–4%. In pregnant women upto 20% may develop fulminant hepatitis E with mortality rate of upto 80% of such cases.

Ans. 81. iii. 1886.

Ans. 82. iii. Doxycycline.

Ans. 83. ii. Japan.

Ans. 84. i. Dead end host for leptospirosis.

Ans. 85. i. Motile.

Ans. 86. iii. Feral swine.

Ans. 87. i. Animals only.
The organisms tend to localize in the reproductive organs of the animals, causing sterility and abortions. They are shed in large numbers in the urine, milk and placental fluid of the infected animals.

Ans. 88. iv. Doxycycline.
A 6 week regimen of doxycycline 200 mg/day administered orally, with the addition of streptomycin 1 gm/day administered intramuscularly for the first 2–3 weeks is effective therapy for adults with most forms of Brucellosis. The WHO recommended treatment regime is a combination of both rifampicin 600–900 mg/day and doxycycline 200 mg/day given orally for 6 weeks.

Ans. 89. ii. Pneumonia.
The most common complications of measles result from involvement of the respiratory tract or the central nervous system (CNS). The most serious complications include blindness, encephalitis, severe diarrhea possibly leading to dehydration, ear infections including otitis media, and severe respiratory infections such as pneumonia, which is the most common cause of death associated with measles.

Ans. 90. i. Single-stranded RNA virus.

Ans. 91. iii. Lifelong.

Ans. 92. iii. 1966.
A live attenuated vaccine against measles has been available since 1966. A number of strains like the Edmonston B strain, Schwarz strain and

Moraten strain are used in vaccine manufacture. The vaccine is extremely effective and safe.

Ans. 93. i. 0.25 ml/kg body weight.
Passive immunization involves the administration of normal human immunoglobulin at a dose: 0.25 ml/kg body weight. The immunoglobulin should ideally be administered within 6 days of exposure. Passive immunization is indicated for vulnerable susceptible household contacts like immune compromised children. HIV infected children must also receive passive immunization, even if they have been vaccinated.

Ans. 94. ii. Togaviridae.
The rubella virus is an enveloped, single-stranded RNA virus of the genus *Rubivirus* from the family Togaviridae.

Ans. 95. ii. 60 nm.

Ans. 96. iii. 10 and 15.
The virus is highly communicable but less so than measles and varicella. As the disease has a large proportion of subclinical cases, they become important factors in disease transmission. Cases are infective from 10 days before to 15 days after onset of rash.

Ans. 97. ii. 18 days.
The incubation period ranges from 12–23 days, with an average of 18 days. Viremia occurs about a week after exposure and leads to viral spread to different organs. A large proportion of cases of postnatal rubella are subclinical. Children suffer from a milder form of the disease as compared to adults. Adults may have prodromal features of fever, malaise and anorexia. Generalized lymphadenopathy and a maculopapular rash are major clinical manifestations.

Ans. 98. iii. 15–18th month.

Ans. 99. iii. Both endemic and epidemic.
Chickenpox occurs in both endemic and epidemic forms in India. There has been a signifi-

cant decline in the incidence and mortality due to chickenpox in countries with widespread pediatric immunization.

Ans. 100. iv. Double-stranded DNA virus.

Ans. 101. ii. Less than 2/100,000.

Ans. 102. iv. History of exposure and clinical features.

The diagnosis of chickenpox is usually based on history of exposure and clinical features such as the characteristic rash. Laboratory confirmation of diagnosis is usually not required except in cases of atypical disease presentation. A Tzanck smear of vesicular fluid, demonstrates multinucleated giant cells and epithelial cells with eosinophilic intranuclear inclusion bodies. The disease can be confirmed by serology but tests usually take very long for diagnosis. Both IgM and IgG tests are available. IgM antibody testing is not considered useful as the tests are neither highly sensitive nor specific. Rising IgG titer from paired acute and convalescent sera are considered evidence of acute infection. Detection of virus, viral antigen or protein can also be done using electron microscopy or PCR. Direct fluorescent antibody (DFA) tests give rapid reliable results.

Ans. 103. iv. All of the above.

The disease is characterized by vesicular eruptions which are typically unilateral and follow a dermatomal distribution. The most commonly involved dermatomes are thoracic and lumbar. Most cases of herpes zoster occur after the age of 50 years or among immunocompromised persons. It is a relatively common complication in HIV-positive persons occurring in 8–11% of patients. The disease may rarely result in permanent neurological damage in the form of cranial nerve palsies or visual impairment following herpes zoster ophthalmia. Nearly 15% of zoster patients have pain or paresthesia in the affected dermatome for several weeks and sometimes permanently (postherpetic neuralgia).

Disseminated, herpes zoster may occur in patients suffering from malignancies, AIDS or other immunocompromised states. Transmission of Varicella zoster virus from herpes zoster patients may cause chickenpox in nonimmune contacts.

Ans. 104. i. Klebs.
The diphtheria bacillus was first described by Klebs in 1883 and was first cultured by Loeffler in a culture medium of his own design in 1884. It is, therefore, known as the "Klebs-Loeffler" bacillus.

Ans. 105. i. Exotoxin.
The most important factor determining virulence of *Corynebacterium diphtheriae* is the exotoxin. The production of exotoxin depends on a lysogenic β phage. Diphtheria exotoxin causes both local and systemic cell destruction. In addition to the exotoxin, cell-wall components such as the O and K antigens are important in the pathogenesis of the disease.

Ans. 106. ii. Faucial infection.
This is the most common site for respiratory diphtheria. The patient has fever, malaise and sore throat. The characteristic feature is the development of a membrane on one or both sides. The membrane may be confined to the tonsils or extend over a larger area including the uvula, soft palate, oropharynx and nasopharynx. The extent of the membrane corresponds with the severity of the symptoms. The membrane is white in color to begin with, but rapidly changes to a gray color. Attempts to remove the membrane result in bleeding. Cases with severe disease develop marked local edema resulting in a "bull neck" appearance and respiratory stridor.

Ans. 107. iii. Laryngeal or tracheobronchial infection.
This is the most severe type of respiratory infection. It usually results from a downward spread of pharyngeal infection. Patients present with cough, hoarseness of voice, respiratory stridor and may even have dyspnea.

Ans. 108. iii. Encapsulated.

Ans. 109. i. 13.

They differ in their agglutination reactions to sera directed against polysaccharide antigens. At least 13 sero groups have been described: A, B, C, D, E, H, I, K, L, W–135, X, Y and Z. Almost all meningococcal infections are caused by 5 sero groups A, B, C, 29E or W – 135.

Ans. 110. iii. A and C.

The predominant sero groups in Asia and Africa are A and C while sero groups B and C are responsible for the majority of cases in Europe and the Americas.

Ans. 111. ii. 3–4 days.

The average incubation period is 3–4 days with a range of 2–10 days. This is also the period of communicability. The bacteria are rapidly eliminated from the nasopharynx after starting antibiotics, usually within 24 hours. Humans are the only reservoir. Both cases and carriers serve as the source of infection.

Ans. 112. iv. Decreased protein concentration.

The diagnosis of meningococcal meningitis is suspected by the clinical presentation and a lumbar puncture showing a purulent spinal fluid. Typical CSF abnormalities in meningitis include the increased pressure (>180 mm water), WBC counts between 10 and 10,000 cells/μL, (predominantly neutrophils), decreased glucose concentration (< 45 mg/dL) and increased protein concentration (> 45 mg/dL).

Ans. 113. ii. Penicillin.

The adult dose of penicillin is 4 million units IV 4 times a day. The pediatric dose is 250,000 units/kg/day given intravenously in divided doses.

Ans. 114. i. Tuberculosis.

Ans. 115. iv. 80%

Ans. 116. ii. Pulmonary tuberculosis

Primary infection occurs on first exposure to tubercle bacilli. Inhaled droplet nuclei are so small that they avoid the mucociliary defences of the bronchi and lodge in the terminal alveoli of the lungs. Infection begins with multiplication of tubercle bacilli in the lungs. This is the *Ghon focus*. Lymphatics drain the bacilli to the hilar lymph nodes. The *Ghon focus* and related hilar lymphadenopathy form the primary complex. Bacilli may spread in the blood from the primary complex throughout the body.

Ans. 117. iv. African.

Tuberculosis has been controlled almost completely in the developed world. Almost all the cases and practically all deaths due to tuberculosis take place in developing countries.

Though the absolute numbers of cases and deaths are the largest in Asia, the rates of disease and deaths are the highest in Africa. South Africa and Nigeria rank first to fifth respectively in terms of absolute numbers of cases. The African Region has the highest incidence rate per capita (363/1,00,000 population).

Ans. 118. iii. India.

Tuberculosis is the biggest public health problem in the country. With 1.8 million cases occurring annually, India accounts for a fifth of the world's new TB cases and 2/3rd of the cases in South-East Asia. This makes India the highest TB burden country in the world. It has been estimated that for the year 2000 there were about 3.8 million bacteriologically positive TB cases in the country. Overall prevalence of infection in India is estimated to be 30% while the annual incidence of infection is estimated to be 1–2%. The prevalence of disease is thought to be 4 per 1000 and the incidence of disease 1.5 per 1000. The prevalence of infection has been found to be increasing with age. The peak age for males is 45–54 years and that for females is 35 years. No rural-urban differences in the rate have been found.

Ans. 119. iii. 3000 droplet nuclei.

Mycobacterium tuberculosis is spread by airborne particles, known as droplet nuclei that can be generated when persons with pulmonary or laryngeal tuberculosis sneeze, cough, speak, or sing. It has been estimated that a cough can generate 3000 droplet nuclei. The same number is generated by a person talking for 5 minutes. Persons who share the same airspace with persons with infectious tuberculosis disease are at greatest risk for infection. Infection occurs when a susceptible person inhales droplet nuclei containing tubercle bacilli and these bacilli become established in the alveoli of the lungs and spread throughout the body. Prolonged household contact with an open case may lead to infection.

Ans. 120. ii. 2+.

Ans. 121. i. 4 H3 R3.

Ans. 122. i. Category I regimen.

Ans. 123. iii. Rifampicin.

RNTCP advocates using a standardized treatment regimen comprising of 6 drugs (kanamycin, ofloxacin, ethionamide, pyrazinamide, ethambutol and cycloserine) during 6–9 months of the intensive phase and 4 drugs (ofloxacin, ethionamide, ethambutol and cycloserine) during the 18 months of the continuation phase for cases of MDR–TB.

Ans. 124. iii. Hong Kong.

The first documented infection of humans with an avian influenza virus occurred in Hong Kong in 1997, when the H5N1 strain caused severe respiratory disease in 18 humans, of whom 6 died.

Ans. 125. i. 1918.

An influenza pandemic is a rare but recurrent event. Three pandemics occurred in the previous century: "Spanish influenza" in 1918, "Asian influenza" in 1957, and "Hong Kong influenza" in 1968. The 1918 pandemic killed an estimated

40–50 million people worldwide. That pandemic, which was exceptional, is considered one of the deadliest disease events in human history.

Ans. 126. iv. Nasopharyngeal aspirate.

Ans. 127. ii. Oseltamivir.

2 drugs (in the neuraminidase inhibitors class), Oseltamivir (commercially known as Tamiflu) and Zanamivir (commercially known as Relenza) can reduce the severity and duration of illness caused by seasonal influenza. The efficacy of the neuraminidase inhibitors depends on their administration within 48 hours after symptom onset. For cases of human infection with H5N1, the drugs may improve prospects of survival, if administered early, but clinical data are limited. The H5N1 virus is expected to be susceptible to the neuraminidase inhibitors.

Ans. 128. iii. Vaccination.

In developing countries, nonmedical interventions may be the main line of defence throughout the first wave of a pandemic. Health education to inform the general public especially small poultry farmers is essential to reduce exposure risk. Stringent sanitary measures and appropriate biosecurity practices should be applied, including the control of human traffic and introduction of birds of unknown disease status into the flock. Carcasses of suspected and confirmed poultry case of influenza should preferably be incinerated or buried deep using lime and soil in the ratio of 1 : 3. The H5N1 avian influenza virus is not transmitted to humans through properly cooked food. The virus is sensitive to heat. Normal temperatures used for cooking (so that food reaches 70°C in all parts) will kill the virus. To date, no evidence indicates that any person has become infected with the H5N1 virus following the consumption of properly cooked poultry or poultry products, even in cases where the food item contained the virus prior to cooking. Poultry and poultry products from areas free of the disease can be prepared and consumed as usual, with no fear of acquiring infection with the H5N1 virus. As a standard precaution, WHO recommends that poultry and poultry products should always be prepared following good hygienic practices, and that poultry meat should be properly cooked.

Ans. 129. iv. China.

As on 15th May 2003, a cumulative total of 7548 probable cases and 573 deaths due to SARS have been reported from 29 countries. The affected areas were : the People's Republic of China (PRC), particularly the Hong Kong Special Administrative Region and the Beijing Municipality, Guangdong, Inner Mongolia, Shanxi, Tianjin, Taiwan Province (China), Toronto (Canada), Singapore (Singapore), India and Manila (Philippines). As of now, China has reported more cases than the rest of the world combined. Currently, there is no known SARS transmission anywhere in the world.

Ans. 130. iii. Andhra Pradesh.

As on 14th May, 2003, 3 probable cases of SARS have been reported from India, one each in West Bengal, Karnataka and Gujarat.

Ans. 131. i. Enveloped RNA virus.

SARS corona virus is an enveloped RNA virus. The SARS virus has fulfilled the Koch's postulates, and it has been successfully cultivated in vitro (in vero cell line) as well as in vivo (experimental infection has been established in monkeys). The genome of the SARS corona virus is somewhat similar to that of other corona viruses, however the detailed sequence data confirm that this SARS corona virus is a previously unrecognized corona virus.

Ans. 132. ii. 48 hours.

The WHO network laboratories have shown that the SARS virus can survive after drying on plastic surfaces for upto 48 hours. The virus can survive in feces for at least 2 days and in urine for upto 24 hours.

Ans. 133. ii. 10.

Detect antibodies in serum of SARS patients 10 days after the onset of illness.

Ans. 134. iv. Prevalence greater than 50%, heavy infection more than 10%.

Based on the prevalence and the intensity of the infection, the communities can be classified into 3 categories—

a. Category I (high) transmission community: Prevalence greater than 50%, heavy infection more than 10%.
b. Category II (medium) transmission community: Prevalence greater than 50%, heavy infection less than 10%.
c. Category III (low) transmission community: Prevalence less than 50%, heavy infection less than 10%.

Ans. 135. ii. Indirect.

Based on their life cycle, STH can be classified into three types:

a. Type 1–Direct: The eggs are embryonated. They hatch and reinfect within 2–3 hours by direct carriage from anal margin to the mouth. Eggs do not reach the soil, and if they do, do not require a period of development there. For example—*Enterobius vermicularis* (threadworm), *Trichuris trichiura* (whipworm).
b. Type 2–Modified direct: Eggs are passed in stools and undergo a period of development in soil to become the infective stage, before being ingested. After ingestion, eggs hatch and release larva which penetrate mucous membrane of stomach and enter circulation and pass up the respiratory tract, enter esophagus, reach intestine and grow into adult. For example—*Ascaris lumbricoides* (roundworm).
c. Type 3–Penetration of the skin: Eggs are passed in the stool to soil. In soil, eggs hatch into larvae which undergo development till they are ready to penetrate the skin. The larvae penetrate the skin, reach circulation and lungs where they penetrate

lungs to reach respiratory tract, enter esophagus, reach small intestine and grow into adult. For example—*Ancylostoma duodenale* (hookworm).

Ans. 136. i. *Wuchereria bancrofti.*
Food borne helminths include a variety of flukes and tapeworms. The notable among these are *Fasciola buski* (intestinal flukes), *Fasciola hepatica* (liver flukes), *Clonorchis sinensis* (liver flukes, Chinese liver fluke, oriental liver fluke), *Paragonimus westermani* (lung flukes), *Taenia saginata* (beef tapeworm) and *Taenia solium* (pork tapeworm).

Ans. 137. iii. Enterobius (threadworm).
Retrograde infection—The eggs laid on perianal skin immediately hatch into infective-stage larvae and migrate through the anus to develop into adult forms in the colon.

Ans. 138. iv. 30,000
The diagnosis is established by the finding of characteristic eggs by a direct microscopical examination of a saline emulsion of stool. An egg count reveals the degree of infection. A count of 30,000 eggs per gram of feces or more is considered as heavy infection.

Ans. 139. ii. Moderate prevalence.

Ans. 140. iv. Pyrantel pamoate.
Pyrantel pamoate given in a single dose of 10 mg/kg body weight is safe as well as effective in pregnancy.

Ans. 141. i. 1 definitive host and 2 intermediate hosts.

Ans. 142. iii. Praziquantel.

Ans. 143. ii. Lung fluke.

Ans. 144. i. Pig.

Ans. 145. ii. *Trichinella spiralis* (trichina worm)

Ans. 146. iv. 1 mg of iron/10,000 ova/gm of feces.
The main consequence of chronic hookworm infection is iron deficiency anemia. Such an

infection can result in a daily loss of 1 mg of iron/10,000 ova/gm of feces, irrespective of the species. Heavy infection may also lead to malabsorption and hypoproteinemia.

Ans. 147. iii. 15%.
In India, the prevalence of amebiasis ranges from 3.5–45% with an average of about 15%.

Ans. 148. iv. Cyst.
The cyst is the infective form of the organism and survives in soil, water, sewage and feces for several days. It is not affected by the routine chlorination of the water but is readily killed if dried, frozen or heated to 55°C or more.

Ans. 149. ii. Man.
The source of infection is the food and drink contaminated with human feces. Contamination of water supplies with raw sewage has been reported to cause epidemics.

Ans. 150. iv. Cecum and ascending colon.
The most common intestinal manifestation of the disease is abdominal discomfort associated with diarrhea which subsequently turns into dysentery. Lower abdominal pain and tenesmus is common and tenderness is present over cecum and colon. Patient may pass 10–12 stools per day. The stools contain little fecal material and consist mainly blood and mucous. Fever is usually absent (fever is common in bacillary dysentery) in amebiasis. Fulminant intestinal infection with severe abdominal pain, high fever and profuse diarrhea is rare. In such cases, patient may develop toxic megacolon.

Ans. 151. ii. Does not affect children.
Amebiasis can occur at any age.

Ans. 152. iv. Patients with AIDS.
The high-risk group includes travellers, migrants, immigrant workers, immunocompromised individuals, prisoners and children in day-care centers. Severe infections occur in very young children,

pregnant women, malnourished and people taking corticosteroids. Patients with AIDS do not have an increased risk of severe infection.

Ans. 153. i. Metronidazole.

Metronidazole is the drug of choice for the treatment of both intestinal amebiasis and amebic liver abscess. It is given in a dose of 750 mg orally or IV three times a day for 5–10 days. Tinidazole 2 gm once a day for 3 days is an alternative to metronidazole. In addition to the above, one of the following luminal amebicides should be prescribed as an adjunctive treatment, either concurrently or sequentially, to destroy *E. histolytica* in the colon:

- Paromomycin 500 mg 3 times a day for 10 days
- Diloxanide furoate 500 mg 3 times a day for 10 days
- Iodoquinol 650 mg 3 times a day for 20 days.

Ans. 154. ii. 10%

Amebiasis occurs worldwide but the majority of the cases are reported from developing countries mainly because of poor hygiene and sanitary conditions. These areas include India, Mexico, Central and South America and countries of Africa and Asia in tropical regions. In developed countries, the affected population is mainly constituted by travellers. At any onetime approximately 10% of the world population is affected by amebiasis. It is the third most common cause of death, after schistosomiasis and malaria, from parasitic diseases.

Ans. 155. ii. 2.

Food safety measures should be taken to protect food and drink from fecal contamination. Food handlers with amebiasis must be excluded from work and should not be permitted back till one stool specimen is negative. In outbreak circumstances, a second consecutive negative stool specimen will be required prior to returning to work.

Ans. 156. iv. Duodenum and upper jejunum.

Giardia lamblia, is a flagellate protozoan parasite of human being. It exists in 2 forms—The trophozoite which inhabits the duodenum and upper part of jejunum and the cyst which exists outside the host and is the form that transmits the infection.

Ans. 157. ii. 12%.

The infection is common among travellers who travel from developed countries to developing countries. Upto 12% of the traveller's diarrhea is said to be because of the giardia infection.

Ans. 158. iv. All.

The aim of the control program is to prevent infections and the ill health resulting from the above conditions through various interventions. Some studies has demonstrated that STD treatment is an important prevention strategy in HIV infection in a general population. The main aims of STD control are:

- To interrupt the transmission of sexually acquired infections.
- To prevent the development of diseases, complications and sequelae.
- To reduce the risk of HIV infection.

These objectives can be achieved by programs through primary prevention directed at reducing the incidence of disease, and through secondary prevention directed at reducing prevalence by shortening the duration of disease, thus minimizing the probability of complications or sequelae.

Ans. 159. iii. Couples in monogamous relationship.

Ans. 160. ii. Description of treatment for different syndromes.

Education should be carried out through lectures, multimedia, flip charts, group or individual discussions and articles in the periodicals/journals/newspapers read by general population. Most of the prevention messages will apply to both

HIV and conventional STDs but the educational messages which specifically relate to STDs will include:

- Though not necessarily practical or desirable, abstinence is the only way to completely prevent STIs.
- Avoid sex with many different partners. The less sexual partners a person has, the lower the risk of infection.
- Sexually transmitted diseases can be avoided to a large extent by practicing safe sex (e.g. using condoms).
- Information that symptoms and signs may not be noticed, particularly in women, until complications appear.
- Description of recognizable signs and symptoms.
- A list of places where STD advice may be obtained (i.e. basic health care services), and where available, categorical STD clinics and voluntary counseling centers.
- Assurance that wherever services are obtained in the public sector privacy, confidentiality and respect are guaranteed.
- Advice on assessing one's personal risk of having acquired an STD, and also that of sexual partner(s). (If the assessment suggests a possibility of STD, attendance for STD advice is indicated).

Ans. 161. iv. All.

Case Detection: It is an essential part of any control program. The usual methods of early case detection are:

a. Screening: Screening of special high risk or vulnerable groups is done for early detection of disease.
b. Contact tracing: The sexual partners of diagnosed patients are identified, located, investigated and treated.
c. Cluster testing: The patients are asked to name other persons of either sex who move in the same socio-sexual environment.

Ans. 162. i. To make a correct diagnosis.

Adequate treatment of patients and their contacts is the mainstay of STD control. Holding patient to ensure complete and adequate treatment is key to effective management. The STI care, should aim to provide the comprehensive case management that includes diagnosis, curative treatment, reduction of risk-taking behavior and the treatment of sexual partners. The objective of case management of patients with STIs is:

- To make a correct diagnosis
- To provide effective treatment
- To reduce/prevent future risk-taking behavior
- To advise on treatment compliance
- To promote and provide condoms
- To ensure sexual partners are notified and appropriately treated.

Ans. 163. iv. All.

Ans. 164. iv. Staphylococcus.

Ans. 165. i. 15–30%.

From 15–30% infants born to HIV-infected mothers are infected before, during, or shortly after birth: treatment of pregnant women results in marked reduction in infant infections.

Ans. 166. iv. Disseminated TB.

An adult or adolescent (>12 years) is considered to have AIDS if a test for HIV antibody is positive, and one or more of the following criteria are present:

a. Weight loss>10% or cachexia, with diarrhea or both, intermittent or constant, for > 1 month.
b. Tuberculosis with weight loss > 10%, or disseminated, miliary, or extrapulmonary tuberculosis.
c. Kaposi's sarcoma.
d. Neurologic impairment preventing independent daily activities.
e. Esophageal candidiasis.
f. Cryptococcal meningitis.
g. Life-threatening or recurrent episodes of pneumonia.
h. Invasive cervical cancer.

Ans. 167. iv. Persistent cough for more than 1 month.

Major signs:
- Weight loss or abnormally slow growth
- Chronic diarrhea for more than 1 month
- Prolonged fever for more than 1 month

Minor signs:
- Recurrent common infections, e.g. ear infection, pharyngitis
- Persistent cough
- Generalized rash
- Oropharyngeal candidiasis
- Generalized lymphadenopathy.

Ans. 168. iii. Prognostic marker.
Absolute CD4 lymphocyte count is most widely used prognostic marker. Process of testing of HIV is done in 5 stages, first is risk assessment of the individual, then is pretest. Counseling in which information about all aspects of disease and its subsequent medical, social and economic impact is given, next informed consent of the patient is taken. And then testing for HIV is done and lastly posttest counseling for both negative and positive subjects.

Ans. 169. ii. Social contact.

Ans. 170. ii. 50/cu mm.
People with healthy immune system usually have counts above 950 CD4 cells/cu mm of blood. The number falls over the course of HIV infection. People with AIDS usually have CD4 cell count below 200/cu mm.

Ans. 171. ii. NNRTI.

Ans. 172. i. Preferably within 1–2 hours.
PEP should be initiated as quickly as possible, preferably within 1–2 hours of exposure and upto 36 hours postexposure.

Ans. 173. iv. All.

Ans. 174. iv. All.

Ans. 175. ii. Conduct routine episiotomies.

Good prenatal care, adequate antiretroviral therapy to the mother and child, cesarean section, and exclusive or no breastfeeding are all associated with decreased transmission of HIV. Even in mothers without chronic therapy for HIV and without prenatal care, antiretroviral agents like zidovudine given through labor and delivery, together with early treatment of the newborn, decrease significantly the risk of transmission. Zidovudine is administered to women during pregnancy, labor and delivery and to their newborns: The rate of HIV transmission is decreased by two-thirds. In addition to the use of ARV drugs, the following obstetric practices will reduce the risk of mother to child transmission:

a. Avoidance of early rupture of membranes
b. Avoidance of routine episiotomies
c. Using nontraumatizing suction cups on vacuum extractors where possible
d. Avoid fetal scalp puncture.

Ans. 176. iv. All.

Monitoring

Testing source: If there is no recent positive or negative serology, a rapid test is preferred, since results should be available in <10 minutes. Standard serologic tests may take 3–7 days, but a negative EIA screening assay is usually available in 24–48 hours and is adequate for the decision to discontinue PEP.

Testing health care worker: HIV serology should be performed at the time of injury, and repeated at 6 weeks, 3 months, and 6 months. Most health care workers who seroconverted had symptomatic acute HIV syndrome, usually 2–6 weeks postexposure.

Caution: The health care worker should be advised to practice safe sex or abstain until serology is negative at 6 months postexposure. The greatest risk is the first 6–12 weeks.

Time: PEP should be initiated as quickly as possible, preferably within 1–2 hours of exposure and upto 36 hours postexposure.

Side effects: For health care workers who receive PEP, about 74% experience side effects, primarily nausea (58%), fatigue (37%), headache (16%), vomiting (16%), or diarrhea (14%). About 53% discontinue treatment before completion of the 4 weeks course due to multiple factors including side effects of drugs. The HCWs should, therefore, be properly briefed on these aspects to ensure compliance.

Ans. 177. i. Hansen's disease.

Ans. 178. i. 10.

A quick random sample survey is done to collect baseline data in the community. Contact surveillance of households with a lepromatous case is recommended for a minimum period of 10 years after case is declared bacteriologically negative.

Ans. 179. ii. 5.

Contact surveillance of households with a lepromatous case is recommended for a minimum period of 5 years in households with a nonlepromatous case from the time of diagnosis of the index case.

Ans. 180. ii. 6 or more lesions.

In 1987, WHO study group endorsed that all the patients showing smear positivity should be classified as having multibacillary leprosy for the purpose of MDT treatment. Same study group in 1993 gave clinical classification into 2 groups:

a. Paucibacillary leprosy (1–5 skin lesions)
b. Multibacillary leprosy (more than 5 skin lesions).

Ans. 181. ii. 48 hours and 21days.

The lepromin test, also called Mitsuda reaction, was first described by the Japanese worker, K Mitsuda in 1916. It is an intradermal immunological test employed to detect CMI and classify the type of disease and to find out the prognosis in a given case. Lepromin is a suspension of lepromatous tissue rich in *M. leprae* in an isotonic solution of sodium chlorides sterilized by heating. The test is performed by injecting intradermally 0.1 ml of lepromin or lepra antigen in the forearm of a patient and the reaction is examined at the end of 48 hours and 21 days.

Ans. 182. i. 6 months.

Ans. 183. i. Clinical.

Ans. 184. i. 5.

The Indian classification is the official classification of the Indian Leprosy Association and most widely used in India. It is clinicobacterial classification and described as under:

a. Indeterminate type: Early cases with one or two vague hypopigmented macules and with and without sensory impairment. Lesions are bacteriologically negative.
b. Tuberculoid type: Cases with one or two well-defined lesions which may be flat or raised, hypopigmented or erythematous and are anesthetic.
c. Borderline type: Cases with four or more lesions which may be flat or raised, well or ill-defined, hypopigmented or erythematous and shows sensory impairment or loss. Bacteriological positivity is variable and if left untreated can progress to lepromatous type.
d. Lepromatous type: Cases with diffuse infiltration or numerous flat or raised lesions, symmetrical without any sensory loss.
e. Pure neuritic type: Cases show nerve involvement but do not have any lesion in skin. Cases are bacteriologically negative.

4 Epidemiology of Noncommunicable Diseases

Ischemic Heart Disease (IHD) SVN: Coronary Heart Disease (CHD): Coronary Artery Disease (CAD)

Q.1. ***The estimated deaths due to IHD in industrialized countries is:***

i. 25–30%
ii. 40–55%
iii. 80–90%
iv. 10–20%

Q.2. ***It is estimated that number of IHD cases in India is around:***

i. 55 million
ii. 15 million
iii. 30 million
iv. 1 million

Q.3. ***The desirable, borderline high and high values of total cholesterol are:***

i. < 200, 200–239, ≥ 240
ii. < 160, 160–180, > 180
iii. < 200, 200–249, > 250
iv. < 180, 181–191, > 192

Q.4. ***The desirable value of HDL cholesterol:***

i. ≤ 30
ii. ≤ 60
iii. ≤ 50
iv. ≤ 40

Q.5. ***The optimal, near optimal, borderline high, high, very high values of LDL cholesterol are:***

i. < 100, 100–129,130–159, 160–189, > 190
ii. < 120, 120–129, 130–159, 160–199, > 200

iii. < 130, 130–159, 160–199, > 200
iv. < 100, 130–159, 160–189, > 190

Q.6. ***Metabolic syndrome does not include*:**

i. WHR > 0.9 for males or > 0.85 for females
ii. Albumin excretion < 20 microgram
iii. Low levels of HDL cholesterol: < 40 mg/dL in men, < 50 mg/dL in women
iv. Elevated blood pressure levels: ≥ 140 mm Hg SBP or ≥ 90 mm Hg DBP

Q.7. ***Atherogenic diet does not include*:**

i. High in total calories, total fat, saturated fats and cholesterol
ii. High in salt and refined sugar
iii. Low in whole grains, cereals, legumes, fruits, vegetables
iv. High in antioxidants

Q.8. ***Not a coronary risk factor*:**

i. Raised nonHDL cholesterol
ii. Raised TC: HDL-C ratio (> 4.5)
iii. Low apolipoprotein A-1
iv. Low apolipoprotein B

Q.9. ***Lower cut-off of BMI for overweight as recommended for Asian populations is*:**

i. > 18.5
ii. > 20.5
iii. > 23
iv. > 24.9

Q.10. ***One of the following is a mode of primary prevention*:**

i. Individual risk prediction charts
ii. Resting ECG using Minnesota Code Criteria
iii. Rose questionnaires
iv. Exercise ECG

Q.11. ***Early diagnosis and treatment of hypertension is _______ mode of prevention for IHD*:**

i. Primordial
ii. Primary

iii. Secondary
iv. Tertiary

Q.12. ***Early diagnosis and treatment of angina is _______ mode of prevention for IHD*:**

i. Primordial
ii. Primary
iii. Secondary
iv. Tertiary

Q.13. ***Early diagnosis and treatment of dyslipidemia is _______ mode of prevention for IHD*:**

i. Primordial
ii. Primary
iii. Secondary
iv. Tertiary

Q.14. ***Not a modifiable coronary risk factor*:**

i. Raised nonHDL cholesterol
ii. Raised TC: HDL-C ratio
iii. Low apolipoprotein A-1
iv. MI in father before 45 years age

Diabetes Mellitus

Q.15. ***Type 1 Diabetes is not characterized by*:**

i. Abrupt onset of severe symptoms
ii. Proneness to ketosis
iii. Onset below 30 years
iv. It comprises upto 40% of all diabetes

Q.16. ***Type 2 Diabetes is not characterized by*:**

i. Comprising 85–90% of all diabetes cases
ii. Quite often detected on a routine screening tests
iii. Diagnosis being often made after 40 years age
iv. Very weak genetic (family history) component

Q.17. ***As per the American Diabetic Association (ADA), a person is said to be diabetic when the plasma fasting glucose is more than or equal to (in mg/dL)*:**

i. 100
ii. 126

iii. 200
iv. 110

Q.18. ***As per the American Diabetic Association (ADA), a person is said to be diabetic when the plasma postprandial glucose is more than or equal to (in mg/dL):***

i. 100
ii. 126
iii. 200
iv. 110

Q.19. ***Drug-induced diabetes is seen in:***

i. Thiazides
ii. Beta blockers
iii. Corticosteroids
iv. All of the above

Q.20. ***Not a risk factor for diabetes:***

i. Increased dietary intake of saturated fat and decreased intake of fiber
ii. Poor maternal nutrition during pregnancy
iii. Stress
iv. High sodium and low potassium intake

Cancer

Q.21. ***Worldwide, the most common cause of death from cancer is that of:***

i. Lung
ii. Oral cavity
iii. Gastric
iv. Liver

Q.22. ***Following is not the characteristic of a cancer:***

i. Clonality
ii. Metastasis
iii. Anaplasia
iv. All of the above

Q.23. ***The most common cancer in Indian women is:***

i. Breast
ii. Cervix

iii. Endometrium
iv. Oral cavity

Q.24. *Match the following*:

1. Aflatoxin	a. Esophageal cancer
2. Ochratoxin A	b. Hepatocellular carcinoma
3. *F. verticillioides* or its toxins	c. Urinary tract cancer
4. Asbestos	d. Lung

Q.25. *Use of combined oral contraceptives accounts for an increase in risk of*:

i. Breast cancer
ii. Ovarian cancer
iii. Endometrial cancer
iv. None

Q.26. *Exposure to benzene causes the following cancer*:

i. Bladder
ii. Lung
iii. Prostate
iv. Leukemia

Q.27. *Smoking is not a known risk factor for which of the following cancer*:

i. Pancreas
ii. Kidney
iii. Bladder
iv. Prostate

Q.28. *At present number of population based cancer registries (PBCRs) in India is*:

i. 5
ii. 6
iii. 7
iv. 4

Q.29. *At present number of hospital-based cancer registries (HBCRs) in India is*:

i. 5
ii. 6
iii. 7
iv. 4

Q.30. ***Match the following cancer with an infection:***

1. Cervix uteri	a. *Schistosoma haematobium*
2. Lymphoid tissues	b. *Helicobacter pylori*
3. Stomach	c. Epstein-Barr virus
4. Urinary system	d. Human papilloma virus

Q.31. ***Cancer not having genetic susceptibility is:***

i. Neurofibromatosis
ii. Breast
iii. Ovarian
iv. All of the above have genetic susceptibility

Q.32. ***Visual inspection with acetic acid (VIA) is a method of screening for:***

i. Oral cavity
ii. Cervix
iii. Gastric
iv. Prostate

Mental Health

Q.33. ***Out of all cases of depression, what percentage is formed by neuropsychiatric illnesses?***

i. 20–30%
ii. 30–40%
iii. 40–50%
iv. 10–20%

Q.34. ***The prevalence rate of mental morbidity in India is:***

i. 25.8/1000
ii. 58.2/1000
iii. 107.6/1000
iv. None of the above

Q.35. ***All of the following are major symptoms of schizophrenia except:***

i. Obsessions
ii. Hallucinations
iii. Delusions
iv. Cognitive symptoms

Q.36. ***Mean onset of age for schizophrenia is higher in which sex:***

i. Males
ii. Females
iii. Equal in both sexes
iv. None of the above

Q.37. ***Neurotic, stress related and somatoform disorders includes which one of the following:***

i. Depression
ii. Obsessive compulsive disorder
iii. Eating disorder
iv. Mental retardation

Chronic Obstructive Pulmonary Diseases

Q.38. ***Which of the following is a diagnostic criteria for COPD?***

i. FEV1 less than 80% of the predicted value
ii. FEV1 less than 90% of the predicted value
iii. FEV1 less than 85% of the predicted value
iv. FEV1 less than 94% of the predicted value

Q.39. ***Mild COPD is characterized by:***

i. FEV1 less than 80% predicted value
ii. FEV1 more than 80% predicted value
iii. FEV1 less than 50% predicted value
iv. FEV1 less than 60% predicted value

Q.40. ***Very severe COPD is characterized by:***

i. FEV1 less than 80% predicted value
ii. FEV1 more than 80% predicted value
iii. FEV1 less than 30% predicted value
iv. FEV1 less than 60% predicted value

Q.41. ***The gold standard for diagnosis and assessment of COPD is:***

i. Chest X-ray
ii. Spirometry
iii. Clinical examination
iv. None of the above

Q.42. ***Most important pharmacotherapy for the management of COPD is:***

i. Bronchodilators
ii. Glucocorticosteroids

iii. Anticholinergics
iv. None of the above

Q.43. ***The most cost-effective intervention to reduce the risk of developing COPD and stop its progression is:***

i. Pharmacotherapy
ii. Better nutrition
iii. Reducing indoor air pollution
iv. Cessation of smoking

Visual Impairment and Blindness

Q.44. ***What percentage of all AIDS patients show evidence of some ocular disease?***

i. 10–20%
ii. 30–40%
iii. 40–70%
iv. 80–100%

Q.45. ***Visual impairment category 3, 4 and 5 is termed as:***

i. Low vision
ii. Blindness
iii. Both
iv. Neither

Q.46. ***Immunization against which particular disease is part of specific protection measures aimed at preventing blindness:***

i. Mumps
ii. Measles
iii. Rubella
iv. Chickenpox

Answers

Ans. 1. i. 25–30%.

Ans. 2. iii. 30 million.

Ans. 3. i. < 200, 200–239, ≥ 240.

Ans. 4. iv. ≤ 40.

Ans. 5. i. < 100, 100–129, 130–159, 160–189, > 190.

Ans. 6. ii. Albumin excretion < 20 microgram.

Ans. 7. iv. High in antioxidants.

Ans. 8. iv. Low apolipoprotein B.

Ans. 9. iii. > 23.

Ans. 10. i. Individual risk prediction charts.

Ans. 11. ii. Primary.

Ans. 12. iii. Secondary.

Ans. 13. ii. Primary.

Ans. 14. iv. MI in father before 45 years age.

Ans. 15. iv. It comprises upto 40% of all diabetes.

Ans. 16. iv. Very weak genetic (family history) component.

Ans. 17. ii. 126.

Ans. 18. iii. 200.

Ans. 19. iv. All of the above.

Ans. 20. iv. High sodium and low potassium intake.

Ans. 21. i. Lung.

Ans. 22. iv. All of the above are characteristics.

Ans. 23. ii. Cervix.

Ans. 24. 1—b, 2—c, 3—a, 4—d.

Ans. 25. i. Breast cancer.

Ans. 26. iv. Leukemia.

Ans. 27. iv. Prostate.

Ans. 28. ii. 6.

Ans. 29. i. 5.

Ans. 30. 1—d, 2—c, 3—b, 4—a

Ans. 31. iv. All of the above have genetic susceptibility.

Ans. 32. ii. Cervix.

Ans. 33. ii. 30–40%.

Ans. 34. ii. 58.2/1000.

Ans. 35. i. Obsessions.

Ans. 36. ii. Females.

Ans. 37. ii. Obsessive compulsive disorder.

Ans. 38. i. FEV1 less than 80% of the predicted value.

Ans. 39. ii. FEV1 more than 80% predicted.

Ans. 40. iii. FEV1 less than 30% predicted.

Ans. 41. ii. Spirometry.

Ans. 42. i. Bronchodilators.

Ans. 43. iv. Cessation of smoking.

Ans. 44. iii. 40–70%.

Ans. 45. ii. Blindness.

Ans. 46. ii. Measles.

5 Demography and Family Health

Q.1. ***According to the demographic cycle, India is in the following phase:***

i. High stationary
ii. Early expanding
iii. Late expanding
iv. Low stationary

Q.2. ***According to Central Registration Act of 1969, birth is to be reported within:***

i. 7 days
ii. 14 days
iii. 10 days
iv. 21 days

Q.3. ***Annual growth rate is between:***

i. Crude birth rate—Crude death rate
ii. Crude birth rate—IMR
iii. Total fertility rate—Death rate
iv. Crude birth rate—Total fertility rate

Q.4. ***Census in India is done every:***

i. 5 years
ii. 10 years
iii. 15 years
iv. 20 years

Q.5. ***The most cost-effective family planning method is:***

i. Vasectomy
ii. Barrier method
iii. IUCD
iv. Oral pills

Q.6. ***The year of "Big Divide" is:***

i. 1900
ii. 1901

iii. 1920
iv. 1921

Q.7. ***As per census 2001 average annual growth rate of India is (in %):***

i. 2.01
ii. 1.93
iii. 1.80
iv. 1.86

Q.8. ***As per census 2001 decadal growth rate of India is (in %):***

i. 21.34
ii. 31.93
iii. 11.80
iv. 9.86

Q.9. ***As per census 2001, the percentage of world's population from India is:***

i. 26
ii. 16
iii. 10
iv. 6

Q.10. ***As per census 2001, lowest populated state of India is:***

i. Kerala
ii. Sikkim
iii. Goa
iv. Nagaland

Q.11. ***The annual growth rate of India presently characterized as:***

i. Slow
ii. Rapid
iii. Very rapid
iv. Explosive

Contraceptive Technology

Q.12. ***In rhythm method for contraception, intercourse is avoided during:***

i. 3–14 days
ii. 5–25 days

iii. 10–28 days
iv. 7–21 days

Q.13. ***In basal body temperature method for contraception, increase in body temperature occurs:***

i. Just before the ovulation
ii. Ovulation period itself
iii. Immediately after ovulation
iv. Menstruation

Q.14. ***The failure rate of cervical mucus method if used correctly is:***

i. 1/HWY
ii. 2/HWY
iii. 3/HWY
iv. 4/HWY

Q.15. ***The failure rate of condom is:***

i. 12–14 HWY
ii. 14–17 HWY
iii. 17–20 HWY
iv. 20–25 HWY

Q.16. ***The active agent in spermicidal jelly is:***

i. 9-Xylenolol
ii. 9-Xylene
iii. 9-Nonoxynol
iv. 9-Nonxylenol

Q.17. ***In Cu T200, 200 signifies:***

i. Weight of Cu in mg
ii. Surface area of Cu in sq mm
iii. Length of Cu wire in mm
iv. Diameter of Cu wire in μm

Q.18. ***The mechanism of action of IUD does not include:***

i. Inducing mild inflammatory changes and foreign body reaction in the endometrium
ii. Incapacitate the sperms and ovum, prevent sperm from fertilizing the ovum
iii. Makes the uterine environment inhospitable for the blastocyst to be implanted
iv. Increases the reverse peristalsis of uterus

Q.19. ***Which of the following IUDs belong to Gp II IUDs?***

i. Cu T200
ii. Lippes loop
iii. Cu T380A
iv. ML-250

Q.20. ***The presence of Cu T in place is checked routinely by:***

i. Feeling the thread coming out of cervical os
ii. Absence of menstruation
iii. Feeling the metal tip in upper part of vagina
iv. None of the above only X-ray can check it

Q.21. ***Which one is not an absolute contraindication for IUD insertion?***

i. Pregnancy
ii. Puerperal sepsis
iii. Anemia
iv. Bleeding P/V of unknown etiology

Q.22. ***Which of the following is not the likely adverse effect of IUD?***

i. Menorrhagia
ii. Metrorrhagia (intermenstrual bleeding)
iii. Polymenorrhea
iv. Anemia

Q.23. ***Single pill of MALA-D contains:***

i. L-norgesterol (LNGL) 0.15 mg and EE 0.03 mg
ii. L-norgesterol (LNGL) 0.03 mg and EE 0.15 mg
iii. D-norgesterol (LNGL) 0.15 mg and EE 0.03 mg
iv. D-norgesterol (LNGL) 0.03 mg and EE 0.15 mg

Q.24. ***Which of the following is not the likely mechanism of action of OCPs?***

i. Inhibition of ovulation by bringing about changes in FSH and LH secretion
ii. By altering the endometrium
iii. By bringing about changes in cervical mucus
iv. Incapacitates sperm

Q.25. ***Which of the following is not the likely adverse effect of OCP?***

i. Menorrhagia
ii. Breast heaviness

iii. Oligomenorrhea
iv. Dysmenorrhea

Q.26. ***The failure rate of OCP is:***

i. 1 HWY
ii. 2–3 HWY
iii. 0.1 HWY
iv. 10 HWY

Q.27. ***Which is not the contraindication for OCP use?***

i. Hyperlipidemia
ii. Cirrhosis of liver
iii. Unexplained vaginal bleeding
iv. Anemia

Q.28. ***Which of the following is most cost-effective method for permanent sterilization?***

i. Vasectomy
ii. Pomeroys tubectomy
iii. Laparoscopic tubectomy
iv. No scalpel vasectomy

Q.29. ***After vasectomy/no scalpel vasectomy, for at least how many months should the couple use alternative temporary method of contraception?***

i. 3 weeks
ii. 3 months
iii. 2 weeks
iv. 2 months

Q.30. ***Emergency contraceptive pill should be used within a maximum period of:***

i. 24 hours
ii. 48 hours
iii. 72 hours
iv. 96 hours

Q.31. ***What is a mini pill?***

i. Pill containing lesser amount of estrogen and progesterone
ii. Once a month pill
iii. Progesterone only pill
iv. Emergency pill

Answers

Ans. 1. iii. Late expanding.

Ans. 2. ii. 14 days.

Ans. 3. i. Crude birth rate – Crude death rate.

Ans. 4. ii. 10 years.

Ans. 5. i. Vasectomy.

Ans. 6. iv. 1921.

Ans. 7. ii. 1.93.

Ans. 8. i. 21.34.

Ans. 9. ii. 16.

Ans. 10. ii. Sikkim.

Ans. 11. iii. Very rapid.

Ans. 12. iv. 7–21 days.

Ans. 13. iii. Immediately after ovulation.

Ans. 14. iii. 3/HWY.

Ans. 15. i. 12–14 HWY.

Ans. 16. iii. 9-Nonoxynol.

Ans. 17. ii. Surface area of Cu in sq mm.

Ans. 18. iv. Increases the reverse peristalsis of uterus.

Ans. 19. iv. ML-250.

Ans. 20. i. Feeling the thread coming out of cervical os.

Ans. 21. iii. Anemia.

Ans. 22. iii. Polymenorrhea.

Ans. 23. i. L-norgesterol (LNGL) 0.15 mg and EE 0.03 mg.

Ans. 24. iv. Incapacitates sperm.

Ans. 25. iv. Dysmenorrhea.

Ans. 26. iii. 0.1 HWY.

Ans. 27. iv. Anemia.

Ans. 28. iv. No scalpel vasectomy.

Ans. 29. ii. 3 months.

Ans. 30. iii. 72 hours.

Ans. 31. iii. Progesterone only pill.

6 Maternal and Child Health

Q.1. ***Which of the following is not included in 'Cleans' in conduct of delivery*:**

i. Clean hands
ii. Clean perineum
iii. Clean cutting and care of the cord
iv. Clean surface of delivery

Q.2. ***In India, majority of deliveries take place at*:**

i. Hospital
ii. Primary health center
iii. Private clinics
iv. Home

Q.3. ***Antenatal care includes*:**

i. Genetic counseling for prospective parents
ii. Spacing of births
iii. Ensuring adequate maternal nutrition
iv. All of the above

Q.4. ***Janani Suraksha Yojana has been started under*:**

i. CSSM
ii. NRHM
iii. MCH
iv. ICDS

Q.5. ***Iron/folic acid tablets are distributed to private doctors for free distribution under which scheme*:**

i. NRHM
ii. CSSM
iii. Janani Suraksha Yojana
iv. Vande Mataram Scheme

Q.6. ***Followings are high-risk antenatal cases except*:**

i. Elderly primi
ii. Preeclampsia

iii. Twin pregnancy
iv. None

Q.7. ***Minimum number of antenatal visits during pregnancy is:***

i. 2
ii. 3
iii. 5
iv. 6

Q.8. ***MMR in India is:***

i. 300/lakh
ii. 400/lakh
iii. 200/lakh
iv. 500/lakh

Integrated Management of Neonatal and Childhood Illnesses (IMNCI)

Q.9. ***General danger signs in a sick child include all except:***

i. Convulsions
ii. Unconsciousness
iii. Inability to breastfeed
iv. Vomiting

Q.10. ***Which of the following is not true of dehydration?***

i. Mild to moderate dehydration can be corrected at home by ORS
ii. ORS solution should be made fresh daily
iii. Breastfeeding should be delayed till dehydration is corrected
iv. Patient should be given as much ORS as he wants

Q.11. ***Young infants in IMNCI guidelines are upto the age of:***

i. 6 months
ii. 1 year
iii. 2 months
iv. 3 months

Q.12. ***For young infants assessment is basically done for all except:***

i. Jaundice
ii. Hypothermia

iii. Diarrhea
iv. Measles

Q.13. ***IMNCI recommendations are upto the age of:***

i. 10 years
ii. 8 years
iii. 7 years
iv. 5 years

Q.14. ***Severe jaundice in a neonate are all except:***

i. Less than 24 hours
ii. More than 7 days
iii. More than 14 days
iv. Yellow discoloration of palms and soles

Q.15. ***In a 6 months old child breathing rate ___________ or more suggests pneumonia:***

i. 40/minute
ii. 50/minute
iii. 60/minute
iv. 70/minute

Q.16. ***Signs for classifying a child as having severe dehydration are all except:***

i. Dry tongue
ii. Sunken eyes
iii. Not able to drink
iv. Lethargic or unconscious

Q.17. ***A case of simple pneumonia is treated with:***

i. Parenteral antibiotics
ii. Oral antibiotics
iii. Referred to hospital
iv. Parenteral antibiotics and referral

Q.18. ***IMNCI approach developed by WHO encompasses following childhood illnesses except:***

i. Measles
ii. Malaria
iii. Diarrhea
iv. Chickenpox

Genetics and Public Health

Q.19. ***The Austrian monk who presented the results of his breeding experiments on garden peas in 1865 was:***

i. James Watson
ii. Gregor Mendel
iii. William Bateson
iv. Johannsen

Q.20. ***The term 'Gene' was coined by:***

i. James Watson
ii. Gregor Mendel
iii. William Bateson
iv. Johannsen

Q.21. ***The double helical structure of DNA was proposed by:***

i. Watson and Crick
ii. Mendel and Wilkins
iii. Bateson and Garrod
iv. Johannsen and Maurice

Q.22. ***How many genes are estimated to be in the human genome?***

i. 50,000
ii. 1,00,000
iii. 1,50,000
iv. 2,00,000

Q.23. ***The process where genetic information is transmitted from DNA to RNA is called:***

i. Processing
ii. Transcription
iii. Translation
iv. Sequencing

Q.24. ***The site for protein synthesis in the cell is the:***

i. Mitochondria
ii. Nucleus
iii. Cytoplasm
iv. Ribosome

Q.25. ***How many amino acids are involved in formation of proteins?***

i. 10
ii. 15

iii. 20
iv. 25

Q.26. ***The triplet of nucleotide bases in mRNA which codes for a particular amino acid is called:***

i. Structural genes
ii. Codon
iii. Control genes
iv. Genome

Q.27. ***The stability of DNA is based on:***

i. Coding
ii. Noncoding
iii. Mutation
iv. DNA repair

Q.28. ***The process of cell division ensures that the human zygote which is a single cell at conception undergoes rapid division leading to cells in an adult:***

i. 104
ii. 1010
iii. 1014
iv. 1020

Q.29. ***Edward's syndrome is:***

i. Trisomy 21
ii. Trisomy 13
iii. Trisomy 18
iv. Trisomy 22

Q.30. ***Patau's syndrome is:***

i. Trisomy 21
ii. Trisomy 13
iii. Trisomy 18
iv. Trisomy 22

Q.31. ***Concordance in monozygotic twins should be greatest when disease onset is early.***

True/False

Q.32. ***Multigenic diseases require a specific environment for their occurrence.***

True/False

Q.33. ***The burden of diseases of genetic etiology in a community is determined by all except:***

i. Gene pool
ii. Breeding pattern
iii. Migration
iv. None

Q.34. ***Chromosomal deletion disorder associated with chromosome 4 is called:***

i. Wolf-Hirschhorn syndrome
ii. Cri-du-chat syndrome
iii. Retinoblastoma
iv. Wilms tumor

Answers

Ans. 1. ii. Clean perineum.

Ans. 2. iv. Home.

Ans. 3. iv. All of the above.

Ans. 4. ii. NRHM.

Ans. 5. iv. Vande Mataram Scheme.

Ans. 6. iv. None.

Ans. 7. ii. Three.

Ans. 8. i. 300/lakh.

Ans. 9. iv. Vomiting.

Ans. 10. iii. Breastfeeding should be delayed till dehydration is corrected.

Ans. 11. iii. 2 months.

Ans. 12. iv. Measles.

Ans. 13. iv. 5 years.

Ans. 14. ii. More than 7 days.

Ans. 15. ii. 50/minute.

Ans. 16. i. Dry tongue.

Ans. 17. ii. Oral antibiotics.

Ans. 18. iv. Chickenpox.

Ans. 19. ii. Gregor Mendel.

Ans. 20. iv. Johannsen.

Ans. 21. i. Watson and Crick.

Ans. 22. ii. 1,00,000.

Ans. 23. ii. Transcription.

Ans. 24. iv. Ribosome.

Ans. 25. iii. 20.

Ans. 26. ii. Codon.

Ans. 27. iv. DNA repair.

Ans. 28. iii. 1014

Ans. 29. iii. Trisomy 18.

Ans. 30. ii. Trisomy 13.

Ans. 31. True

Ans. 32. False

Ans. 33. iv. None

Ans. 34. i. Wolf-Hirschhorn syndrome.

7 Nutrition in Public Health

Q.1. ***Who coined the term 'vitamin'?***

i. McCollum
ii. Funk
iii. Hopkins
iv. James Lind

Q.2. ***A teacher will be classified as a:***

i. Sedentary worker
ii. Moderate worker
iii. Heavy worker
iv. Average worker

Q.3. ***A 'safety margin' of + 2 SD is not incorporated for the RDA of:***

i. Energy
ii. Fats
iii. Water-soluble vitamins
iv. Fat-soluble vitamins

Q.4. ***Which of the following diseases is most notorious to prove fatal in combination with malnutrition?***

i. Tetanus
ii. Anemia
iii. Measles
iv. Diarrhea

Q.5. ***Choosing what type of food to eat in a household is the function of the:***

i. Family
ii. Government
iii. Community
iv. Any of the above

Micronutrients: The Vitamins

Q.6. ***Which of the following will help you increase the iron absorption from diet?***

i. Nicotinic acid
ii. Ascorbic acid
iii. Pantothenic acid
iv. Folic acid

Q.7. ***Which of the following is not a source of beta carotene?***

i. Green vegetable
ii. Potato
iii. Liver
iv. Papaya

Q.8. ***Which of the following is not known to have an antioxidant effect?***

i. Vitamin A
ii. L-ascorbic acid
iii. Alpha-tocopherol
iv. Phylloquinone

Q.9. ***Which of the following does not fall under 'xerophthalmia'?***

i. Conjunctival xerosis
ii. Corneal xerosis
iii. Retinal xerosis
iv. Lachrymal xerosis

Q.10. ***Which of these is available only from animal sources:***

i. Vitamin B_{12}
ii. Vitamin B_1
iii. Vitamin B_6
iv. Vitamin B_2

The Micronutrients: Minerals

Q.11. ***Which of the following iron sources falls under the category of nonheme iron?***

i. Jaggery
ii. Meat
iii. Eggs
iv. Milk

Q.12. ***Calcium homeostasis is maintained by:***

i. T_3 and T_4
ii. Vitamin D and parathyroid hormone
iii. Phosphorus and magnesium
iv. Calcitonin and bone matrix

Q.13. ***Ideal sodium potassium ratio should be:***

i. Not specified
ii. 1:1
iii. 1:2
iv. 2:1

Q.14. ***Which of the following does not fall under 'IDD'?***

i. Cretinism
ii. Mongolism
iii. Deaf-mutism
iv. Infertility

Q.15. ***Which of these is not a constituent of metalloenzymes?***

i. Copper
ii. Zinc
iii. Iron
iv. Nickel

Major Foods and their Nutritive Value

Q.16. ***The highest content of niacin is present in:***

i. Jaggery
ii. Groundnuts
iii. Pistachio
iv. Milk

Q.17. ***Yellow-orange fruits and vegetables are rich in:***

i. Carotenes
ii. Vitamin D
iii. B complex vitamins
iv. Zinc

Q.18. ***Food item with highest protein content is:***

i. Groundnuts
ii. Meat
iii. Soya bean
iv. Fish

Q.19. ***Egg is a poor source of vitamin:***

i. A
ii. B
iii. C
iv. D

Q.20. ***Jaggery is a rich source of:***

i. Carotene and thiamine
ii. Zinc and iron
iii. Iron and carotene
iv. Sugar and proteins

Nutritional Requirements of Special Groups: Mothers, Children and the Elderly

Q.21. ***Which of the following is not true regarding diet for the elderly?***

i. Their poor dentition restricts their food intake
ii. The zeal to cook and eat goes down
iii. Their food requirement is about half that of a robust young adult
iv. There is not enough research to accurately predict RDA for elderly

Q.22. ***Which of the following is not true regarding diet during lactation?***

i. Energy requirement during lactation is higher than during pregnancy
ii. Iron requirement during lactation is higher than during pregnancy
iii. Vitamin C requirement during lactation is higher than during pregnancy
iv. Vitamin A requirement during lactation is higher than during pregnancy

Q.23. ***Higher need of vitamin A during pregnancy can be met by all except:***

i. Carrots
ii. Cod liver oil capsules
iii. Extra egg whites
iv. Extra milk

Q.24. ***Which of the following is true about diet during pregnancy?***

i. Salt intake must be minimized to prevent edema
ii. Diet before pregnancy has no bearing on health of neonate
iii. Strict weight control helps minimize childbirth complications
iv. One extra meal per day is recommended during pregnancy

Q.25. ***Which of these is not true for weaning?***

i. Weaning means gradually replacing breast milk with other foods
ii. It should be started at 1 year of age
iii. One must start weaning with fruit juices and cow's milk
iv. Infant is more vulnerable to infections during this period

Nutritional Deficiency Diseases

Q.26. ***Jelliffe gave the ___________ term in year 1959:***

i. PEM
ii. PCM
iii. Food gap
iv. Marasmus

Q.27. ***The highest number (60.3%) of underweight children (under 3 years) is reported from:***

i. Bihar
ii. Madhya Pradesh
iii. Uttar Pradesh
iv. Jharkhand

Q.28. ***In ______________ child is 'skin and bones' owing to loss of subcutaneous tissue:***

i. Kwashiorkor
ii. Stunting
iii. Nephrotic syndrome
iv. Marasmus

Q.29. *Term 'Kwashiorkor' was introduced by __________ into modern medicine*:

i. Cicely Williams
ii. Jelliffe
iii. Ghai
iv. Barbar Mc Klintok

Q.30. *Anemia contributes to ______ % of all maternal deaths*:

i. 10
ii. 20
iii. 5
iv. 30

Q.31. *It is generally believed that spinach is a 'very good' source of iron. But the fact is that it is a poor source as it contains only__________ mg iron per 100 gm*:

i. 5.5
ii. 6.0
iii. 1.1
iv. 10.0

Q.32. *Apart from India, other South East Asian country/ies prone to iodine deficiency is/are _______________* :

i. Myanmar
ii. Thailand
iii. Sri Lanka
iv. All of these

Q.33. *It is estimated that the total population at risk in India is about ________ million and ________ million are estimated to suffer from IDD*:

i. 20 and 7
ii. 100 and 35
iii. 40 and 14
iv. 200 and 70

Q.34. *For infants less than 1year old or less than 8 kg weight, the dose of vitamin A used is ________* :

i. 4,00,000 IU (110 mg) of retinol palmitate (oil miscible vitamin A) administered orally for 2 days
ii. 2,00,000 IU (110 mg) of retinol palmitate (oil miscible vitamin A) administered orally for 2 days

iii. 1,00,000 IU (110 mg) of retinol palmitate (oil miscible vitamin A) administered orally for 2 days
iv. 2,00,000 IU (110 mg) of retinol palmitate (oil miscible vitamin A) administered orally for 1 day

Q.35. ***Hb threshold (mg%) to label anemia in nonpregnant women (≥15.00 years) is ____________:***

i. 3.0
ii. 12.0
iii. 10.5
iv. 11.0

Q.36. ***For a patient to suffer from dental fluorosis, the fluorine intake through water has to be at least:***

i. > 1.5 ppm
ii. 1.0 ppm
iii. 0.5 ppm
iv. 5.0 ppm

Q.37. ***Poker Back, Rose Thorn appearance on chest X-ray and genu valgum are features of ____________:***

i. Hypervitaminosis D
ii. Hypervitaminosis A
iii. Skeletal fluorosis
iv. Congenital hypercalcemia

Food Hygiene and Sanitary Regulation of Eating Establishments

Q.38. ***Which is true for mushrooms?***

i. It is a nutritious food
ii. Some mushrooms could cause food borne disease
iii. Some mushrooms could cause food poisoning
iv. All of the above

Q.39. ***Which of the following is generally not a source of food borne diseases?***

i. Dust
ii. Skin infection
iii. Home preserved food
iv. Fruits

Q.40. ***Pasteurization destroys:***

i. All pathogenic organisms
ii. Some pathogenic organisms
iii. Most pathogenic organisms
iv. No pathogenic organisms

Q.41. ***Which of these insecticides is relatively safe for kitchen use?***

i. Abate
ii. Sodium hypochlorite
iii. Baygon
iv. Pyrethrum

Q.42. ***Which of these is the ideal method of disposing off solid refuse from slaughter house?***

i. Incineration
ii. Land fill
iii. Sell it off to a contractor and get some money
iv. Chemical treatment

Nutritional Programs in India

Q.43. ***Midday meal program offers:***

i. Half of daily protein and one-third of calorie requirement
ii. Half of daily protein and half of calorie requirement
iii. One-third of daily protein and half of calorie requirement
iv. One-third of daily protein and one-third of calorie requirement

Q.44. ***To a child under 3 years of age, ICDS provides:***

i. 300 kcal energy and 8–10 gm protein
ii. 300 kcal energy and 16–20 gm protein
iii. 500 kcal energy and 8–10 gm protein
iv. 500 kcal energy and 16–20 gm protein

Q.45. ***In rural areas, the administrative unit for the location of ICDS project is:***

i. Gram panchayat
ii. Community development blocks
iii. District headquarter
iv. Primary health center

Q.46. ***Which of the following is not run by the ministry of health and family welfare?***

i. Prophylaxis against nutritional anemia
ii. Vitamin A prophylaxis program
iii. Iodine deficiency disorders control program
iv. ICDS program

Q.47. ***Which of these is not carried out at the anganwadi center?***

i. Supplementary nutrition
ii. Nonformal preschool education
iii. Immunization
iv. Nutrition and health education

Nutritional Assessment and Surveillance of a Community

Q.48. ***All can indicate nutritional status except:***

i. Fall in weight
ii. Falling hair
iii. Failure to gain height
iv. Flag sign

Q.49. ***All are signs of PEM except:***

i. Flag sign
ii. Unilateral pedal edema
iii. Low weight for age
iv. Dermatoses

Q.50. ***Stunting is _________ weight for height but _________ height for age:***

i. Normal: low
ii. Low: normal
iii. Low: low
iv. High: low

Q.51. ***Acute malnutrition may be indicated by:***

i. Stunting
ii. Wasting
iii. Stunting and wasting
iv. All of the above

Q.52. ***Which of these is not true for nutritional surveillance?***

i. It is an ongoing process
ii. It can be used as a nutritional survey technique

iii. It is a close scrutiny of events related to nutritional changes
iv. It provides timely warning for action

Food Processing, Food Adulteration, Food Additives, Preservatives, Food Toxicants and Food Fortification

Q.53. ***Vanilla essence is a food*:**

i. Additive
ii. Fortificant
iii. Supplement
iv. Toxicant

Q.54. ***Which of the following is not a mycotoxin*?**

i. Aflatoxin
ii. Sanguinarine
iii. Deoxynivalenol
iv. Fumonisin

Q.55. ***PFA Act was enacted in the year*:**

i. 1950
ii. 1954
iii. 1962
iv. 1986

Q.56. ***_______ can take a food sample under the PFA act*:**

i. Consumer
ii. Health inspector
iii. Anyone authorized under the gazette
iv. Any of the above

Q.57. ***_________ are not to be used for preservation of foods*:**

i. Irradiation
ii. Bacteria
iii. Antibiotics
iv. Antioxidants

Nutrition during Special Situations: Disasters, Fairs and Festivals, Community Feeding of Children

Q.58. ***At an average ____________ kcal/person should be catered for planning food aid during disaster*:**

i. 2100
ii. 1850

iii. 2400
iv. 2800

Q.59. ***Water must be stored at the rate of _________ liter for drinking and_______ liter for cooking (per day):***

i. 1,1
ii. 2,2
iii. 2,3
iv. 3,2

Q.60. ***One metric tonne grains are sufficient to feed _________ males/day in a disaster situation:***

i. 2100
ii. 1850
iii. 1000
iv. 1500

Q.61. ***In a disaster situation the aims of therapeutic feeding includes all except:***

i. Medical treatment of severely malnourished
ii. Nutritional treatment of severely malnourished
iii. Reduce infant/child deaths
iv. Treat cases of infections

Q.62. ***Community feeding of children is undertaken in all except:***

i. ICDS program
ii. Midday meal program
iii. Balwadi program
iv. School health program

Answers

Ans. 1. ii. Funk.

Ans. 2. i. Sedentary worker.

Ans. 3. i. Energy.

Ans. 4. iii. Measles.

Ans. 5. i. Family.

Ans. 6. ii. Ascorbic acid.

Ans. 7. iii. Liver.

Ans. 8. iv. Phylloquinone.

Ans. 9. iv. Lachrymal xerosis.

Ans. 10. i. Vitamin B_{12}.

Ans. 11. i. Jaggery.

Ans. 12. ii. Vitamin D and parathyroid hormone.

Ans. 13. ii. 1:1.

Ans. 14. ii. Mongolism.

Ans. 15. iv. Nickel.

Ans. 16. ii. Groundnuts.

Ans. 17. i. Carotenes.

Ans. 18. i. Groundnuts.

Ans. 19. iii. C.

Ans. 20. iii. Iron and carotene.

Ans. 21. iii. Their food requirement is about half that of a robust young adult.

Ans. 22. ii. Iron requirement during lactation is higher than during pregnancy.

Ans. 23. iii. Extra egg whites.

Ans. 24. iv. One extra meal per day is recommended during pregnancy.

Ans. 25. ii. It should be started at 1 year of age.

Ans. 26. ii. PCM.

Ans. 27. ii. Madhya Pradesh.

Ans. 28. iv. Marasmus.

Ans. 29. i. Cicely Williams.

Ans. 30. ii. 20%.

Ans. 31. iii. 1.1.

Ans. 32. iv. All of these.

Ans. 33. iv. 200 and 70.

Ans. 34. iii. 1,00,000 IU (110 mg) of retinol palmitate (oil miscible vitamin A) administered orally for 2 days.

Ans. 35. ii. 12.0.

Ans. 36. i. > 1.5 ppm.

Ans. 37. iii. Skeletal fluorosis.

Ans. 38. iv. All of the above.

Ans. 39. iv. Fruits.

Ans. 40. iii. Most pathogenic organisms.

Ans. 41. iv. Pyrethrum.

Ans. 42. i. Incineration.

Ans. 43. i. Half of daily protein and one-third of calorie requirement.

Ans. 44. i. 300 kcal energy and 8–10 gm protein.

Ans. 45. i. Gram panchayat.

Ans. 46. ii. Vitamin A prophylaxis program.

Ans. 47. iii. Immunization.

Ans. 48. ii. Falling hair.

Ans. 49. ii. Unilateral pedal edema.

Ans. 50. i. Normal: low.

Ans. 51. ii. Wasting

Ans. 52. ii. It can be used as a nutritional survey technique.

Ans. 53. i. Additive.

Ans. 54. ii. Sanguinarine.

Ans. 55. ii. 1954.

Ans. 56. iv. Any of the above.

Ans. 57. iii. Antibiotics.

Ans. 58. i. 2100.

Ans. 59. ii. 2,2.

Ans. 60. ii. 1850.

Ans. 61. iv. Treat cases of infections.

Ans. 62. iv. School health program.

8 Physical and Biological Environmental Effect on Health

Adverse Effects of Extreme Hot Environment

Q.1. ***For every additional kilogram of load being carried, how much of additional heat will be produced, when walking at ordinary pace:***

i. 1 kcal/hour
ii. 2 kcal/hour
iii. 3 kcal/ hour
iv. 4 kcal/hour

Q.2. ***All the following are important aspects which determine the dissipation of metabolic heat, in terms of the clothing being worn except:***

i. Insulation
ii. Radiance
iii. Permeability
iv. Absorption

Q.3. ***Globe thermometer is used to measure:***

i. Relative humidity
ii. Ambient temperature
iii. Radiant heat
iv. Air velocity

Q.4. ***Oxford index is dependent on:***

i. DBT
ii. WBT
iii. DBT and WBT
iv. None of the above

Q.5. ***Which is the most commonly used index of thermal stress?***

i. DBT
ii. WBGT

iii. WBT
iv. Oxford

Q.6. ***A good sunscreen ointment should have a sun-protection factor (SPF) of at least, to be able protect against both UVA and UVB rays, when going out in the sun:***

i. 10
ii. 15
iii. 20
iv. 25

Q.7. ***Acclimatization to heat takes how many days?***

i. 2–6 days
ii. 6–10 days
iii. 10–14 days
iv. 14–18 days

Health Aspects of Extreme Cold Environment

Q.8. ***Age group which is most vulnerable to effects of cold is?***

i. <5 years
ii. 5–65 years
iii. >65 years
iv. i and iii

Q.9. ***Which of the following is a nonfreezing cold injury (NFCI)?***

i. Frost bite
ii. Trench foot
iii. Hypothermia
iv. Frost nip

Q.10. ***What is the core body temperature in severe hypothermia?***

i. <28°C
ii. <29°C
iii. <30°C
iv. <31°C

Q.11. ***The normal core (rectal) temperature of normal healthy humans is:***

i. 36°–36.5°C
ii. 36.5°–37°C
iii. 37°–37.5°C
iv. 37.5°–38°C

Q.12. ***The basic principle of management in hypothermia is:***

i. Quick warming of the "core" without causing simultaneous vasodilation of the periphery
ii. Quick warming of the "periphery"
iii. Quick warming of the "core" with simultaneous vasodilation of the periphery
iv. None of the above

Q.13. ***In frost bite, local warming is done by placing the affected part in a warm water bath at:***

i. 36°–38°C
ii. 38°–40°C
iii. 40°–42°C
iv. 42°–44°C

Q.14. ***Treatment in trench foot consists of keeping the affected part at what environmental temperature, while keeping rest of the body warm:***

i. 14°–18°C
ii. 18°–22°C
iii. 22°–26°C
iv. 26°–30°C

Q.15. ***About ____ hours of exposure to ____ °C is needed to cause cold injury:***

i. 5 hours, –10°C
ii. 10 hours, –10°C
iii. 10 hours, –5°C
iv. 5 hours, –5°C

Water Supply

Q.16. ***Which of the following is considered an adequate water supply/head/day in urban areas?***

i. 50–100 liter
ii. 100–150 liter
iii. 150–200 liter
iv. 200–250 liter

Q.17. ***The purest water in nature is from:***

i. Lakes
ii. Springs

iii. Rains
iv. Ponds

Q.18. ***Salt concentration in sea water is:***

i. 1.5%
ii. 2%
iii. 3.5%
iv. 5%

Q.19. ***Ground water has the following advantages:***

i. Likely to be free from pathogenic organisms
ii. Usually requires no treatment
iii. Supply is likely to be certain even during dry season
iv. Likely to be hard

Q.20. ***Guinea worm disease was a health problem where there were:***

i. Dug wells
ii. Artesian wells
iii. Tube wells
iv. Step wells

Q.21. ***Which one of the following is not a waterborne disease?***

i. Kala-azar
ii. Poliomyelitis
iii. Giardiasis
iv. Roundworm

Q.22. ***The vital layer of the slow sand filter is also known as:***

i. Superficial layer
ii. Sand bed layer
iii. Schmutzdecke
iv. Chemical layer

Q.23. ***The disinfecting action of chlorine is mainly due to:***

i. Chloride atom
ii. Hypochlorous acid
iii. Chloride ion
iv. Hypochlorite ion

Q.24. ***Action of chlorine is maximum when water pH is around:***

i. 3

ii. 5
iii. 7
iv. 9

Q.25. ***Chlorination does not affect in normal doses*:**

i. Salmonella
ii. Polio
iii. Shigella
iv. HIV

Excreta Disposal

Q.26. ***The depth of the water seal is*:**

i. 2 cm
ii. 2 inches
iii. 20 inches
iv. 20 cm

Q.27. ***Septic tank uses*:**

i. Aerobic digestion
ii. Anaerobic digestion
iii. Both
iv. None

Q.28. ***Which is not a method of secondary treatment of sewage*?**

i. Trickling filter method
ii. Activated sludge method
iii. Screening
iv. Sludge treatment

Q.29. ***In immediate aftermath of disaster, displaced population can use this method*:**

i. Open defecation
ii. Water carriage system
iii. Biogas method
iv. Communal aqua privy

Q.30. ***Oxidation pond works on*:**

i. Aerobic principle during night and anaerobic during day
ii. Aerobic principle during day and anaerobic during night

iii. Aerobic in both day and night
iv. Anaerobic in both day and night

Disposal of Solid Wastes

Q.31. ***Waste paper is an example of*:**

i. Refuse
ii. Rubbish
iii. Garbage
iv. None

Q.32. ***A method of selecting depressed areas or creating artificial trenches where waste matter is thrown and compacted with a layer of earth on top of it is*:**

i. Manure pit
ii. Controlled tipping
iii. Burial
iv. Dumping

Q.33. ***Bangalore method of composting is a type of*:**

i. Aerobic
ii. Anaerobic
iii. Both
iv. None

Q.34. ***Bangalore method of refuse disposal is not recommended for population above*:**

i. 100,000
ii. 200,000
iii. 300,000
iv. 400,000

Q.35. ***Dual disposal of nightsoil and solid waste is seen in*:**

i. Manure pit
ii. Controlled tipping
iii. Composting
iv. Sanitary landfill

Q.36. ***The method of solid waste disposal which is not ideal/ feasible for rural setup is*:**

i. Manure pit
ii. Biogas plant

iii. Burial
iv. Mechanical composting

Management of Biomedical Wastes

Q.37. ***The percentage of biomedical waste generated in a hospital which is nonhazardous is:***

i. 85%
ii. 50%
iii. 25%
iv. 15%

Q.38. ***The quantity of waste generated in a hospital in developed countries is (in kg/bed/day):***

i. 10–15
ii. 5–10
iii. 1–5
iv. >30

Q.39. ***According to the categories of biomedical waste, waste sharps come under which category?***

i. 3
ii. 4
iii. 5
iv. 6

Q.40. ***According to the categories of biomedical waste liquid waste comes under which category?***

i. 8
ii. 7
iii. 5
iv. 6

Q.41. ***According to the categories of biomedical waste incineration ash comes under which category?***

i. 8
ii. 7
iii. 9
iv. 10

Q.42. ***The recommended treatment option for disposal of biomedical wastes with color coding of black is:***

i. Secured landfill
ii. Incineration
iii. Chemical disinfection
iv. None

Q.43. ***Category of biomedical wastes that is not color coded as black*:**

i. 5
ii. 8
iii. 9
iv. 10

Housing and Ventilation

Q.44. ***As per the housing standards recommended by The Environmental Hygiene Committee, subsoil water should be below (in feet)*:**

i. 2
ii. 5
iii. 10
iv. 20

Q.45. ***As per the housing standards recommended by The Environmental Hygiene Committee, height of the roof should not be less than (in feet)*:**

i. 2
ii. 5
iii. 10
iv. 20

Q.46. ***The minimum floor area in a house required for one person should be (in sq ft)*:**

i. 100
ii. 200
iii. 250
iv. 50

Q.47. ***The minimum cubic space in a house required for one person should be (in cu ft)*:**

i. 100
ii. 200

iii. 250
iv. 500

Q.48. ***In a house, window area should be _________ of floor area*:**

i. 1/5th
ii. 2/5th
iii. 1/3rd
iv. 1/2nd

Q.49. ***The recommended number of air changes in living room should be ______ (per hour)*:**

i. 1–2
ii. 2–3
iii. 3–4
iv. 4–5

Environmental Pollution: Air, Soil, Noise and Radiological Pollution

Q.50. ***The main greenhouse gas which is largely contributing to global warming is*:**

i. Carbon dioxide
ii. Methane
iii. Nitrous oxide
iv. Fluorocarbons

Q.51. ***Kyoto protocol is an international agreement which deals with*:**

i. Radioactive pollution
ii. Soil pollution
iii. Emission of greenhouse gases
iv. Noise pollution

Q.52. ***Bhopal Tragedy of 1984 was due to a toxic chemical called*:**

i. Methyl cyanide
ii. Methyl isocyanate
iii. Methyl iso chloride
iv. None of the above

Q.53. ***Soiling index is an index to measure*:**

i. Radioactive pollution
ii. Soil pollution

iii. Air pollution
iv. Water pollution

Q.54. ***The Chernobyl disaster was a major nuclear reactor accident in the Chernobyl Nuclear Power Plant in the Soviet Union occurred in the year:***

i. 1982
ii. 1986
iii. 1989
iv. 1990

Answers

Ans. 1. ii. 2 kcal/hour.

Ans. 2. ii. Radiance.

Ans. 3. iii. Radiant heat.

Ans. 4. iii. DBT and WBT.

Ans. 5. ii. WBGT.

Ans. 6. ii. 15.

Ans. 7. iii. 10–14 days.

Ans. 8. iv. i and iii.

Ans. 9. ii. Trench foot.

Ans. 10. i. <28°C.

Ans. 11. iii. 37°–37.5°C.

Ans. 12. i. Quick warming of the "core" without causing simultaneous vasodilation of the periphery.

Ans. 13. iii. 40°–42°C.

Ans. 14. ii. 18°–22°C.

Ans. 15. ii. 10 hours, –10°C.

Ans. 16. ii. 100–150 liter.

Ans. 17. iii. Rains.

Ans. 18. iii. 3.5%.

Ans. 19. iv. Likely to be hard.

Ans. 20. iv. Step wells.

Ans. 21. i. Kala-azar.

Ans. 22. iii. Schmutzdecke.

Ans. 23. ii. Hypochlorous acid.

Ans. 24. iii. 7.

Ans. 25. ii. Polio.

Ans. 26. i. 2 cm.

Ans. 27. iii. Both.

Ans. 28. iii. Screening.

Ans. 29. i. Open defecation.

Ans. 30. ii. Aerobic principle during day and anaerobic during night.

Ans. 31. ii. Rubbish.

Ans. 32. ii. Controlled tipping.

Ans. 33. ii. Anaerobic.

Ans. 34. i. 100,000.

Ans. 35. iii. Composting.

Ans. 36. iv. Mechanical composting.

Ans. 37. i. 85%.

Ans. 38. iii. 1–5.

Ans. 39. ii. 4.

Ans. 40. i. 8.

Ans. 41. iii. 9.

Ans. 42. i. Secured landfill.

Ans. 43. ii. 8.

Ans. 44. iii. 10.

Ans. 45. iii. 10.

Ans. 46. i. 100 sq ft.

Ans. 47. iv. 500.

Ans. 48. i. 1/5th.

Ans. 49. ii. 2–3.

Ans. 50. i. Carbon dioxide.

Ans. 51. iii. Emission of greenhouse gases.

Ans. 52. ii. Methyl isocyanate.

Ans. 53. iii. Air pollution.

Ans. 54. ii. 1986.

9 Public Health Administration and Community Health Care in India

Organization of Health Care in India

Q.1. ***According to the national health policy, one subcenter for the hilly areas covers a population of*:**

i. 3000
ii. 5000
iii. 1000
iv. 4000

Q.2. ***All are grassroot workers except*:**

i. Anganwadi workers
ii. Traditional birth attendants
iii. Village health guide
iv. Health assistants

Q.3. ***A female multipurpose worker should be able to detect all of the following except*:**

i. Anemia
ii. Renal disease
iii. Hydramnios
iv. Malpresentation

Q.4. ***Which is true about community health center*:**

i. It covers a population of 1 lakh
ii. It has 60 beds with specialties in surgery, medicine and gynecology
iii. Community health officer is selected with a minimum of 5 years of exposure
iv. New medical post of community health officer is created

Q.5. ***One PHC should be present in hilly areas for every*:**

i. 10,000 people
ii. 20,000 people

iii. 30,000 people
iv. 50,000 people

Q.6. ***Guideline for selection of village health guide are all except:***

i. They should be permanent resident of local community
ii. They should have minimum formal education at least upto 10th standard
iii. Acceptable to all sections of society
iv. They should be able to spare at least 2–3 hours daily for community health work

Q.7. ***A dai is trained for:***

i. 30 working days
ii. 90 working days
iii. 4 months
iv. 6 months

Q.8. ***Government trains a health guide from a village:***

i. Every year
ii. Once in 3 years
iii. Once in 5 years
iv. Only once

Q.9. ***Which is not a duty of a traditional birth attendant?***

i. Aseptic delivery
ii. Health education
iii. Injection of tetanus toxoid
iv. Registration of birth

Q.10. ***The minimum number of beds recommended for CHC by IPHS is:***

i. 30
ii. 35
iii. 40
iv. 60

Q.11. ***Health assistants visit subcenter/health workers once in every:***

i. Week
ii. 2 weeks

iii. 3 weeks
iv. Month

Q.12. ***One health assistant (male) is entrusted with the task of supervision of____ subcenters:***

i. 2–3
ii. 5–6
iii. 7–8
iv. Only 2

Q.13. ***Which is false regarding ASHA?***

i. Provided in each village in the ratio of 1/1000 population
ii. A primary resident of the village with formal education upto class IV
iii. Preferably in the age group of 25–45
iv. Selected by the Gram Sabha

Reports of Health Committees

Q. 14. ***Quarantine act was passed in_______ :***

i. 1840
ii. 1825
iii. 1852
iv. 1882

Q.15. ***Bhore committee was formed in_______ :***

i. 1943
ii. 1934
iii. 1948
iv. 1938

Q.16. ***According to Bhore committee each PHC cater for_______ population:***

i. 20,000
ii. 40,000
iii. 25,000
iv. 30,000

Q.17. ***Which committee recommended a basic health worker per 10,000 population?***

i. Bhore committee
ii. Mudaliar committee

iii. Chadha committee
iv. Kartar Singh committee

Q.18. ***Which committee recommended 'No private practise' for government doctor?***

i. Mudaliar committee
ii. Chadha committee
iii. Kartar Singh committee
iv. Jungalwalla committee

Q.19. ***Rural health scheme was based on recommendation of which committee:***

i. Srivastav committee
ii. Chadha committee
iii. Kartar Singh committee
iv. Jungalwalla committee

Q.20. ***Which committee proposed a PHC per 50,000 population with 16 subcenters, each covering a population of 3000–3500?***

i. Mudaliar committee
ii. Chadha committee
iii. Kartar Singh committee
iv. Jungalwalla committee

Q.21. ***Which committee suggested constitution of an All India Health Service in the pattern of Indian Administrative Service?***

i. Mudaliar committee
ii. Chadha committee
iii. Kartar Singh committee
iv. Jungalwalla committee

Q.22. ***Which committee recommended establishment of country-wide cader of basic rural doctors consisting of trained paraprofessionals to extend comprehensive health care delivery to rural community?***

i. Shivaraman committee
ii. Chadha committee
iii. Kartar Singh committee
iv. Jungalwalla committee

Health Planning Process in India

Q.23. ***The 3 major divisions of planning commission are all except:***

i. Program advisors
ii. General secretariat
iii. Technical divisions
iv. Executive division

Q.24. ***All are the subsectors of health in planning commission except:***

i. Water supply and sanitation
ii. Medical education, training and research
iii. Indigenous systems of medicine
iv. Agriculture

Q.25. ***Broad objectives of 5 year plan are:***

i. Control and eradication of major communicable diseases of public health importance
ii. Strengthening basic rural health services by establishing subcenters and primary health centers
iii. Population control
iv. All of the above

Q.26. ***One of the following is not the strategies of 11th plan:***

i. To increase aggregate spending on health by the center and the states
ii. The contribution of the private sector in providing primary, secondary, and tertiary services
iii. To establish medical colleges in rural sectors of country
iv. Health as a right for all citizens is the goal

Q.27. ***11th plan will strive towards:***

i. Accelerate GDP growth from 8–10% and then maintain at 10% in the 12th plan in order to double per capita income by 2016–17
ii. Raise the sex ratio for age group 0–6 to 935 by 2011–12 and to 950 by 2016–17
iii. Attain WHO standards of air quality in all major cities by 2011–12
iv. All of the above

Community-related Policies in India

Q.28. ***World Health Assembly at Alma Ata launched movement known as "Health for All (HFA) by 2000 AD" in the year:***

i. 1988
ii. 1998
iii. 1978
iv. 1983

Q.29. ***The remarkable success of NHP 1983 includes elimination of:***

i. Leprosy
ii. Kala-azar
iii. Filariasis
iv. All of the above

Q.30. ***Noteworthy initiatives under the National Health Policy 2002 includes all except:***

i. Comprehensive primary health care services
ii. Noninvolvement of health volunteers
iii. Well worked out referral system
iv. Integrated network of evenly spread specialty and superspecialty services

Q.31. ***Important health related targets for the eleventh 5 year plan (2007–2012) are:***

i. Reducing maternal mortality ratio (MMR) to 1/1,000 live births
ii. Reducing infant mortality rate (IMR) to 28/1,000 live births
iii. Reducing total fertility rate to 2.1
iv. All of the above

Q.32. ***The immediate/ short-term objectives of NPP 2000 are:***

i. To address the unmet needs for contraception
ii. Strengthen health care infrastructure, and health personnel
iii. Provide integrated service delivery for basic reproductive and child health care
iv. All of the above

Q.33. *The major strategies under NPP 2000 include all except:*

i. Empowering women for improved health and nutrition
ii. Meeting the unmet needs for family welfare services
iii. Providing medical facilities to users from overseas
iv. Focus on underserved population groups

Important National Health Programs

Q.34. *Which of the following is true with respect to goals of RCH - II?*

i. IMR< 45/1000
ii. MMR< 100/100000
iii. Both of the above
iv. None of the above

Q.35. *The long-term objective of RCH-II is to achieve a stable population by:*

i. 2045
ii. 2050
iii. 2015
iv. 2055

Q.36. *Centchroman (nonsteroidal contraceptive) has been developed by:*

i. Indian Institute of Population Sciences
ii. National Institute of Health and Family Welfare
iii. All India Institute of Medical Sciences
iv. Central Drug Research Laboratory, Lucknow

Q.37. *Reducing MMR < 200/100000 is a goal of:*

i. National Health Policy 2002
ii. National Population Policy
iii. Tenth 5 year plan
iv. RCH-II

Q.38. *Home visits for postnatal care for mother and newborn under RCH-II are done on:*

i. Day 2 and 5
ii. Day 3 and 7

iii. Day 1 and 3
iv. Day 3 and 5

Q.39. ***Which of the following is not a critical element of first referral unit in RCH-II?***

i. Availability of surgical interventions
ii. Newborn care
iii. Blood storage facility on a 24 hour basis
iv. Easy accessibility

Q.40. ***A total number of ________ tablets of iron with folic acid are given to a pregnant woman by health worker:***

i. 100
ii. 70
iii. 150
iv. 200

Q.41. ***Under National Nutritional Anemia Prophylaxis Program the strength of iron and folic acid in tablets is:***

i. 60 mg elemental iron and 0.5 mg folic acid
ii. 100 mg of elemental iron and 0.5 mg folic acid
iii. 100 mg of elemental iron and 0.1 mg folic acid
iv. 60 mg elemental iron and 0.1 mg folic acid

Q.42. ***Janani Suraksha Yojana (JSY) aims at reducing maternal and neonatal mortality rate by:***

i. Promoting institutional delivery
ii. Health education
iii. Distribution of iron and folic acid tablets to the mothers
iv. All of the above

Q.43. ***Under IMNCI the pink color chart refers to a treatment at:***

i. Outpatient facility
ii. Home management
iii. Give injection/oral drops
iv. Urgent referral

Q.44. ***The objective of national program for prophylaxis against blindness in children due to vitamin A deficiency is to decrease the prevalence of vitamin A deficiency to:***

i. 0.1%
ii. 0.2%

iii. 0.3%
iv. 0.001%

Q.45. ***The objective of national program for prophylaxis against blindness in children due to vitamin A deficiency is being implemented through*:**

i. RCH program
ii. National program for control of blindness
iii. UIP
iv. None of the above

Q.46. ***Goal of national tuberculosis control program is*:**

i. To eradicate TB
ii. To decrease the transmission of TB
iii. To treat all sputum +ve patients
iv. To decrease the incidence of TB to such a low level that is no longer a major public health problem

Q.47. ***Which of the following is an objective of RNTCP?***

i. To achieve at least 70% cure rate of the newly diagnosed sputum smear-positive TB patients
ii. To detect at least 85% of new sputum smear-positive patients after the first goal is met
iii. To achieve at least 85% cure rate of the newly diagnosed sputum smear-positive TB patients
iv. Both (i) and (iii)

Q.48. ***Which of the following is not a component of DOTS ?***

i. Political and administrative commitment
ii. Systematic monitoring and accountability
iii. Supervised treatment to ensure the right treatment
iv. Health education

Q.49. ***Which of the following statement is false?***

i. Duration of intensive phase of category I is 8 weeks
ii. Duration of continuation phase of category II is 22 weeks
iii. Duration of intensive phase of category II is 12 weeks
iv. None of the above

Q.50. ***The total number of doses in category II is:***

i. 78 doses
ii. 102 doses
iii. 108 doses
iv. 76 doses

Q.51. ***Which of the following antitubercular drug is bacteriostatic?***

i. Streptomycin
ii. Ethambutol
iii. INH
iv. Rifampicin

Q.52. ***DOTS plus strategy is for treatment of:***

i. HIV with TB
ii. Malaria with TB
iii. MDR TB
iv. All of the above

Q.53. ***Drug used in chemoprophylaxis of TB is:***

i. INH
ii. Rifampicin
iii. Both of the above
iv. None of the above

Q.54. ***Under NAMP, radical treatment of falciparum malaria is given for:***

i. 1 day
ii. 5 days
iii. 7 days
iv. 14 days

Q.55. ***All of the following statements about NAMP are true except:***

i. MBER should be equal to fever rate of the month in the community
ii. Trends in SPR can be utilized for predicting epidemic situations in the area
iii. Annual blood examination rate is calculated from the number of slides examined per 100 cases of fever
iv. For calculating ABER and MBER the denominator is common

Q.56. ***Function of FTD is best denoted by:***

i. Diagnosis of cases + spraying
ii. Collection of slides + treatment of fever
iii. Only treating fever cases
iv. Treatment + slide collection + spraying

Q.57. ***Which of the following diseases are not included under NVBDCP?***

i. Malaria
ii. Japanese encephalitis
iii. Viral encephalitis
iv. Dengue

Q.58. ***Choice of insecticide for kala-azar elimination under NVBDCP is:***

i. Malathion
ii. Chlorine
iii. Malathion + DDT
iv. DDT

Q.59. ***A person wants to visit a malaria endemic area of low level chloroquine resistant falciparum malaria. The best chemo-prophylaxis is:***

i. Chloroquine
ii. Proguanil + chloroquine
iii. Sulfadoxin + pyrimethamine
iv. Mefloquine

Q.60. ***A malaria survey is conducted in 50 villages having a population of 1 lakh. Out of 20000 slides examined, 500 turned out to be MP positive. The SPR is:***

i. 20%
ii. 5%
iii. 25%
iv. 0.4%

Q.61. ***Which of the following is an indicator for operational efficacy?***

i. API
ii. ABER
iii. AFI
iv. SPR

Q.62. ***Antimalarial month is:***

i. April
ii. May
iii. September
iv. June

Q.63. ***Which of the following statements is false?***

i. Lymphatic filariasis has been targeted for elimination in 2015
ii. Strategy for elimination is by Annual Mass Drug Administration of DEC for 5 years or more
iii. Children less than 2 years are not included in Annual Mass Drug Administration
iv. DEC is safe in pregnancy

Q.64. ***Which one of the following strategies is aimed at AIDS control in India?***

i. Detection and treatment of AIDS cases in the community
ii. Detection and isolation of HIV infected persons in the community
iii. Immune prophylaxis of the risk groups
iv. Community education behavioral change

Q.65. ***AIDS was first detected in India in the year:***

i. 1975
ii. 1981
iii. 1986
iv. 1991

Q.66. ***Which of the following is not true about National AIDS Control Program?***

i. Sentinel surveillance methodology have adopted
ii. Community based screening for prevalence of HIV taken up
iii. Early diagnosis and treatment of STD is a major strategy to control spread of HIV
iv. Formulating guidelines for blood banks donors and dialysis units

Q.67. ***National Leprosy Eradication Program was started in:***

i. 1949
ii. 1955

iii. 1973
iv. 1983

Q.68. ***Elimination in leprosy stands for:***

i. Reduce the number of cases to < 1/10,000 population
ii. Reduce the number of cases to < 1/1000 population
iii. No case of leprosy in a region for 5 years
iv. 100% treatment of all cases

Q.69. ***Which one of the following statements is not correct regarding National Leprosy Eradication Program (NLEP):***

i. Multibacillary leprosy treatment is recommended for 1 year
ii. Skin smear examination is done for classification into paucibacillary and multibacillary
iii. Special action project for elimination of leprosy is for rural areas
iv. Surveillance for 2 years for a treated case of paucibacillary leprosy to be carried out

Q.70. ***India was declared 'Guinea worm disease free' in the year:***

i. 1996
ii. 2000
iii. 2001
iv. 2002

Q.71. ***National Mental Health Program was started in:***

i. 1992
ii. 1983
iii. 1994
iv. 1985

Q.72. ***Which of the following is not a component of AFP surveillance?***

i. Case notification
ii. Case in laboratory investigation
iii. Outbreak response and active search in community
iv. Attaining high routine immunization

Q.73. ***Which of the following is not a strategy for achieving polio eradication?***

i. Attaining high routine immunization
ii. National Immunization Days (NIDs)

iii. Surveillance of acute flaccid paralysis (AFP)
iv. None of the above

Q.74. *National Mental Health Program is:*

i. Vertical program
ii. Integrated program
iii. None of the above
iv. All of the above

Q.75. *National Cancer Control Program was started in:*

i. 1976
ii. 1986
iii. 1970
iv. 1992

Q.76. *Under National Cancer Control Program, oncology wings were sanctioned to:*

i. Regional cancer institutes
ii. District hospital
iii. Medical college hospitals
iv. Voluntary agencies treating cancer patients

Q.77. *National Cancer Registry Program (NCRP) was started by:*

i. Ministry of Health and Family Welfare
ii. Indian Council of Medical Research
iii. Collaboration of (i) and (ii)
iv. None of the above

Q.78. *The goal of NIDDCP is:*

i. To reduce the prevalence of iodine deficiency disorders below 10% in the entire country by 2012 AD
ii. To reduce the prevalence of iodine deficiency disorders below 5% in the entire country by 2012 AD
iii. To reduce the prevalence of iodine deficiency disorders below 10% in the entire country by 2010 AD
iv. None of the above

Q.79. *The best indicator for monitoring the impact of iodine deficiency disorders control program is:*

i. Prevalence of goiter among school children
ii. Urinary iodine levels among pregnant women

iii. Neonatal hypothyroidism
iv. Iodine level in soil

Q.80. ***Which one of the following is not a target disease under vision 2020 'The Right to Sight':***

i. Refractive error
ii. Trachoma
iii. Corneal blindness
iv. Diabetic retinopathy

Q.81. ***Safe strategy in vision 2020 is for which eye condition:***

i. Trachoma
ii. Cataract
iii. Onchocerciasis
iv. Childhood blindness

Q.82. ***Vision 2020 'The right to sight' includes all except:***

i. Trachoma
ii. Epidemic conjunctivitis
iii. Cataract
iv. Onchocerciasis

Q.83. ***ICDS is running under:***

i. Ministry of Health and Family Welfare
ii. Ministry of Women and Child Development
iii. Collaboration of both of above
iv. None of the above

Answers

Ans. 1. i. 3000.

Ans. 2. iv. Health assistants.

Ans. 3. ii. Renal disease.

Ans. 4. i. It covers a population of 1 lakh.

Ans. 5. ii. 20,000 people.

Ans. 6. ii. They should have minimum formal education at least upto 10th standard.

Ans. 7. i. 30 working days.

Ans. 8. ii. Once in 3 years.

Ans. 9. iii. Injection of tetanus toxoid.

Ans. 10. i. 30.

Ans. 11. i. Week.

Ans. 12. ii. 5–6.

Ans. 13. ii. A primary resident of the village with formal education upto class IV.

Ans. 14. ii. 1825.

Ans. 15. i. 1943.

Ans. 16. ii. 40,000.

Ans. 17. iii. Chadha committee.

Ans. 18. iv. Jungalwalla committee.

Ans. 19. i. Srivastav committee.

Ans. 20. iii. Kartar Singh committee.

Ans. 21. i. Mudaliar committee.

Ans. 22. i. Shivaraman committee.

Ans. 23. iv. Executive division.

Ans. 24. iv. Agriculture.

Ans. 25. iv. All of the above.

Ans. 26. iii. To establish medical colleges in rural sectors of country.

Ans. 27. iv. All of the above.

Ans. 28. iii. 1978.

Ans. 29. iv. All of the above.

Ans. 30. ii. Noninvolvement of health volunteers.

Ans. 31. iv. All of the above.

Ans. 32. iv. All of the above.

Ans. 33. iii. Providing medical facilities to users from overseas.

Ans. 34. ii. MMR< 100/100000.

Ans. 35. i. 2045.

Ans. 36. iv. Central Drug Research Laboratory, Lucknow.

Ans. 37. iii. Tenth 5 year plan.

Ans. 38. ii. Day 3 and 7.

Ans. 39. iv. Easy accessibility.

Ans. 40. i. 100.

Ans. 41. ii. 100 mg of elemental iron and 0.5 mg folic acid.

Ans. 42. i. Promoting institutional delivery.

Ans. 43. iv. Urgent referral.

Ans. 44. iii. 0.3%.

Ans. 45. i. RCH program.

Ans. 46. iv. To decrease the incidence of TB to such a low level that is no longer a major public health problem.

Ans. 47. iii. To achieve at least 85% cure rate of the newly diagnosed sputum smear-positive TB patients.

Ans. 48. iv. Health education.

Ans. 49. ii. Duration of continuation phase of category II is 22 weeks.

Ans. 50. ii. 102 doses.

Ans. 51. ii. Ethambutol.

Ans. 52. iii. MDR TB.

Ans. 53. i. INH.

Ans. 54. ii. 5 days.

Ans. 55. iii. Annual blood examination rate is calculated from the number of slides examined per 100 cases of fever.

Ans. 56. ii. Collection of slides + treatment of fever.

Ans. 57. iii. Viral encephalitis.

Ans. 58. iv. DDT.

Ans. 59. ii. Proguanil + chloroquine.

Ans. 60. iii. 25%.

Ans. 61. ii. ABER.

Ans. 62. iv. June.

Ans. 63. iv. DEC is safe in pregnancy.

Ans. 64. iv. Community education behavioral change.

Ans. 65. iii. 1986.

Ans. 66. ii. Community based screening for prevalence of HIV taken up.

Ans. 67. iv. 1983.

Ans. 68. i. Reduce the number of cases to < 1/10,000 population.

Ans. 69. ii. Skin smear examination is done for classification into paucibacillary and multibacillary.

Ans. 70. iii. 2001.

Ans. 71. i. 1992.

Ans. 72. iv. Attaining high routine immunization.

Ans. 73. iv. None of the above.

Ans. 74. ii. Integrated program.

Ans. 75. i. 1976.

Ans. 76. iii. Medical college hospitals.

Ans. 77. iii. Collaboration of (i) and (ii).

Ans. 78. i. To reduce the prevalence of iodine deficiency disorders below 10% in the entire country by 2012 AD.

Ans. 79. iii. Neonatal hypothyroidism.

Ans. 80. iv. Diabetic retinopathy.

Ans. 81. i. Trachoma.

Ans. 82. ii. Epidemic conjunctivitis.

Ans. 83. ii. Ministry of Women and Child Development.

10 Health Systems and Policies

An Introduction to Health Systems

Q.1. ***The total share of health costs of the government towards provision of free health care in India today is:***

i. 17%
ii. 7%
iii. 37%
iv. 50%

Q.2. ***The following is not a method of financing health care systems:***

i. Direct or out-of-pocket payments
ii. General taxation
iii. Social health insurance
iv. None of the above

Q.3. ***The type of health planning which refers to the planned use of power controlled by an individual or organization to force other individuals and organizations to use their own resources in accordance with their plans is:***

i. Dispersed
ii. Focused
iii. Central
iv. None

Social Marketing

Q.4. ***Which of the following is true about social marketing?***

i. Meets identified needs and wants of target market segment
ii. Aims to make a profit by serving the interests of target market

iii. Marketing of products/services mostly through ideas
iv. Marketing of ideas and concepts rather than tangible products

Q.5. ***Social marketing aims to broadly bring about the following changes except:***

i. Cognitive changes among people
ii. Behavior changes among people
iii. Price value changes of that particular product
iv. Changes in false beliefs of an individual

Q.6. ***All of the following are the elements of commercial marketing which are also used in social marketing except:***

i. Product
ii. Place
iii. Price
iv. None of the above

Q.7. ***The accurate identification of the group or individual who is not doing what they should be doing, in terms of health related behavior is known as:***

i. Marketing analysis
ii. Market segmentation
iii. Commercial marketing
iv. None of the above

Q.8. ***Social marketing can be used for:***

i. Health education
ii. Behavior change
iii. Combating many major fatal diseases, especially in children, that can be prevented by vaccination and nutrition
iv. All of the above

Disaster Management

Q.9. ***All of the following are examples of natural disasters except:***

i. Meteorological disasters
ii. Topological disasters
iii. Accidents
iv. Biological disasters

Q.10. ***All of the following are elements of disaster management, except*:**

i. Disaster treatment
ii. Disaster preparedness
iii. Disaster response
iv. Disaster recovery

Q.11. ***Measures aimed at reducing the impact of a natural or man-made disaster on a nation or community, is collectively known by the term*:**

i. Disaster response
ii. Disaster mitigation
iii. Disaster recovery
iv. Disaster prevention

Q.12. ***Relief, rehabilitation and reconstruction are essential components of*:**

i. Disaster mitigation
ii. Disaster response
iii. Both of the above
iv. None of the above

Q.13. ***Overwhelming number of severe injuries which require extensive care, when compare to other disasters, take place in*:**

i. Flooding
ii. Tidal waves
iii. High winds
iv. Earthquakes

Q.14. ***All of the following factors influence the transmission of communicable diseases after natural disasters, except*:**

i. Damage to public utilities
ii. Population movements
iii. Interruption in public health services
iv. Social reactions

Q.15. ***The nodal peripheral unit for providing medical relief in times of disasters, will be*:**

i. Subcenter
ii. Anganwadi

iii. Primary health center
iv. District hospital

Q.16. ***At the district level, the CMO (Chief Medical Officer) will be the chief executive of the disaster management cell.***

Yes/No.

Q.17. ***Among the following choices, the most appropriate one while constructing toilets in disaster scenario, will be:***

i. 1 waterless toilet/25 women
ii. 1 waterless toilet/25 men
iii. 1 waterless toilet/35 women
iv. 1 waterless toilet/45 men

Q.18. ***While considering factors for proper accommodation of homeless persons in disaster situation, the distance from the site to the water point should be not more than:***

i. 50 meters
ii. 100 meters
iii. 150 meters
iv. 250 meters

Q.19. ***Sufficient water of low quality is better than very little water of high quality, in disaster scenarios.***

Yes/No

Q.20. ***While locating water points during times of disasters, if the water points are from ground sources, no sanitation facilities should be definitely not closer than a distance of:***

i. 50 meters
ii. 100 meters
iii. 10 meters
iv. 30 meters

Q.21. ***The ratio of taps to persons as recommended by the United Nations High Commissioner for Refugees (UNHCR), especially in setting of disasters, is:***

i. One tap/100–150 people
ii. One tap/200–250 people
iii. One tap/250–300 people
iv. One tap/50–100 people

Q.22. ***The maximum permissible weight of solid waste that can be collected in a single container, (i.e. weight of a single container, when full), is:***

i. 20–25 kg
ii. 30–35 kg
iii. 40–45 kg
iv. 50–55 kg

Q.23. ***The mean energy requirement per person per day, that has to be catered for by provision of appropriate food, at times of disasters, is:***

i. 2500 kcal
ii. 2000 kcal
iii. 2100 kcal
iv. 2300 kcal

Q.24. ***Mass vaccination campaigns against one of the following diseases would be imperative and helpful in times of disasters:***

i. Typhoid
ii. Cholera
iii. Scrub typhus
iv. Measles

Health Care Financing

Q.25. ***The most important institution and agreement regulating International trade regime at present is:***

i. Free Trade Agreements (FTA)
ii. Doha Declaration
iii. UN Central Products Classification System (UNCPC)
iv. World Trade Organization (WTO)

Q.26. ***The most controversial provisions TRIPS are related to:***

i. Patent protection
ii. Trademark
iii. Copyrights
iv. Industrial designs

Q.27. ***Members "shall not be obliged to, implement in their domestic law more extensive protection than required by this agreement". This is enshrined in which article of TRIPS?***

i. 1
ii. 2

iii. 3
iv. 4

Q.28. ***In 2001, WTO Ministerial Conference endorsed the same approach for the implementation of TRIPS patent provisions at the domestic level in:***

i. Johannesburg
ii. New Delhi
iii. Doha
iv. New York

International Health

Q.29. ***WHO came into force in?***

i. 1942
ii. 1948
iii. 1952
iv. 1945

Q.30. ***World health day is celebrated on:***

i. 24th Oct
ii. 1st Dec
iii. 7th April
iv. 1st Jan

Q.31. ***The administrative and organizational headquarter of UNICEF is at:***

i. Geneva
ii. New York
iii. Rome
iv. Paris

Q.32. ***The administrative and organizational headquarter of UNESCO is at:***

i. Geneva
ii. New York
iii. Rome
iv. Paris

Q.33. ***The FAO was founded in:***

i. 1945
ii. 1942

iii. 1948
iv. 1950

Q.34. ***The administrative and organizational headquarter of ILO is at:***

i. Geneva
ii. New York
iii. Rome
iv. Paris

Q.35. ***The organization which provides expert advice, training and grant support to accomplish MDGs is:***

i. UNICEF
ii. UNDP
iii. UNESCO
iv. UNFPA

Q.36. ***The world's largest international source of funding for population and reproductive health programs is:***

i. UNICEF
ii. UNDP
iii. UNESCO
iv. UNFPA

Q.37. ***The founder of International Red Cross and Red Crescent Movement is:***

i. Rockfeller
ii. Philip Russel
iii. Henry Dunant
iv. None

Q.38. ***Agency which has been supporting the National Tuberculosis Control Program of India is:***

i. IRCS
ii. SIDA
iii. DANIDA
iv. UNICEF

Q.39. ***IHR was completely revised recently in:***

i. 2005
ii. 2007
iii. 2009
iv. 2004

Answers

Ans. 1. i. 17%.

Ans. 2. iii. Social health insurance.

Ans. 3. iv. None.

Ans. 4. iv. Marketing of ideas and concepts rather than tangible products.

Ans. 5. iii. Price value changes of that particular product.

Ans. 6. iv. None of the above.

Ans. 7. ii. Market segmentation.

Ans. 8. iv. All of the above.

Ans. 9. iii. Accidents.

Ans. 10. i. Disaster treatment.

Ans. 11. ii. Disaster mitigation.

Ans. 12. ii. Disaster response.

Ans. 13. iv. Earthquakes.

Ans. 14. iv. Social reactions.

Ans. 15. iii. Primary health center.

Ans. 16. No.

Ans. 17. i. 1 waterless toilet/25 women.

Ans. 18. iii. 150 meters.

Ans. 19. Yes.

Ans. 20. iv. 30 meters.

Ans. 21. ii. One tap/200–250 people.

Ans. 22. i. 20–25 kg.

Ans. 23. iii. 2100 kcal.

Ans. 24. iv. Measles.

Ans. 25. iv. World Trade Organization (WTO).

Ans. 26. i. Patent protection.

Ans. 27. i. 1.

Ans. 28. iii. Doha.

Ans. 29. ii. 1948.

Ans. 30. iii. 7th April.

Ans. 31. ii. New York.

Ans. 32. iv. Paris.

Ans. 33. i. 1945.

Ans. 34. i. Geneva.

Ans. 35. ii. UNDP.

Ans. 36. iv. UNFPA.

Ans. 37. iii. Henry Dunant.

Ans. 38. iii. DANIDA.

Ans. 39. i. 2005.

11 Social, Behavioral and Communication Sciences

Principles of Sociology in Health Care

Q.1. ***Kuppuswamy's scale is based on the following variables except*:**

i. Education
ii. Occupation
iii. Income
iv. Housing

Q.2. ***According to Kuppuswamy's scale, total score for upper middle class is*:**

i. 11–15
ii. 16–25
iii. 26–29
iv. 29–31

Q.3. ***According to Kuppuswamy's scale, total score for upper lower class is*:**

i. 11–15
ii. 16–25
iii. 26–29
iv. 5–10

Q.4. ***The socio-economic scale developed for rural set up is*:**

i. Kuppuswamy
ii. Pareek
iii. Prasad
iv. None of the above

Q.5. ***The following are social security measures against fear and want except*:**

i. ESI scheme
ii. Old age pension
iii. Housing
iv. Life insurance

Family Health History and Individual Medico-social History Taking

Q.6. ***All are true about "Family Registration Number" except:***

i. This is a unique number
ii. No two families would have the same number
iii. May be given by the central government
iv. May be developed by the health care providing unit

Q.7. ***Following dates should be written on the cover except:***

i. The date on which one of the family members were vaccinated
ii. The date on which the folder was updated, since some individual member of the family came in contact with the health care system
iii. The date on which the folder was last updated as a part of the regular survey
iv. The date on which the folder was opened

Q.8. ***Immunization status is recorded in:***

i. Vital statistics record sheet
ii. Sheet for sociodemographic details
iii. Summary-sheet
iv. Sheet for record of housing and environmental sanitation

Q.9. ***Special Health Record Sheets include all except:***

i. Under 5 health card
ii. School-age child health record card
iii. Postnatal health care card
iv. Ration card

Q.10. ***For effective medicosocial case taking one should:***

i. Not maintain good eye contact
ii. Touch patients appropriately
iii. Not discuss patients' personal concerns
iv. Not give patient undivided attention

Q.11. ***In KAP, "P" stands for:***

i. Prevention
ii. Practice

iii. Psychoemotional state
iv. Physical factor

Q.12. ***"SWOT" analysis stand for all except:***

i. Strength
ii. Weakness
iii. Opportunities
iv. Treatment

Q.13. ***Health care services for the family should be assessed in terms of all except:***

i. Availability
ii. Accessibility
iii. Affordability
iv. Accountability

Q.14. ***Socio-economic status according to Kuppuswamy or Prasad scale is calculated under which broad heading:***

i. Social factors in the family
ii. Physical factors in the family
iii. Psychoemotional factors in the family
iv. Factors in the workplace

Q.15. ***Physical factors in the family include all except:***

i. Total number of family members
ii. Housing
iii. Water supply
iv. Nutrition

Q.16. ***Family support system includes:***

i. Financial support
ii. Physical support
iii. Emotional support
iv. All of the above

Q.17. ***Immediate community consists of:***

i. Village
ii. District
iii. State
iv. Country

Q.18. ***Factors in the immediate community include all except:***

i. Community organization
ii. Strength of "we" feeling

iii. Interaction between family members
iv. Cohesiveness between the families in the community

Q.19. ***"Major strengths" of a case can be worked out by analyzing:***

i. Social diagnosis
ii. Social pathology
iii. Psychoemotional state
iv. Support systems

Q.20. ***Plan of management and social therapy includes all except:***

i. Medical management
ii. Giving money
iii. Disability limitation
iv. Emotional support

Health Education

Q.21. ***Which of the following is not a one way communication:***

i. Symposium
ii. Lecture
iii. Group discussion
iv. Stage show

Q.22. ***The best method of health instruction is:***

i. Providing reading assignments
ii. Organizing film show
iii. Setting an example
iv. Giving lectures

Q.23. ***The best way of teaching an urban women about ORS is:***

i. Lecture
ii. Flash cards
iii. Role play
iv. Demonstration

Q.24. ***Receiver's false beliefs are a ______________ type of barrier in communication.***

i. Physiological
ii. Environmental

iii. Cultural
iv. Psychological

Q.25. ***The method which is generally more effective among the following in changing human behavior is:***

i. Counseling
ii. Focus group discussion
iii. Mass media
iv. A series of lectures

Planning, Implementation and Evaluation of Health Education Programs

Q.26. ***Which of the following is not part of situational analysis?***

i. Analyzing the community backdrop
ii. Analysis of community health status
iii. Analysis of community health care system
iv. Defining target communities

Q.27. ***Which of the following is not a part of community diagnosis:***

i. Defining target communities
ii. Defining major health problems
iii. Defining felt needs
iv. Defining the premises

Q.28. ***The aspects considered for outcome evaluation does not include:***

i. Relevance
ii. Adequacy
iii. Process
iv. Resources

Q.29. ***The correct order of following steps is:***

1. Assemble the planning group/co-ordination council
2. Consolidating data on knowledge, attitudes and behaviors
3. Resource analysis
4. Reconfirming the program goals, enunciating the educational goals and the objectives (pick up your choice from one of 1, 2, 3, or 4 as follows:

i. 1, 2, 4, 3

ii. 2, 1, 4, 3
iii. 2, 1, 3, 4
iv. 1, 2, 3, 4

Q.30. ***The best method for health education on treatment of diarrhea/ORS use for urban slum population is:***

i. Lecture
ii. Demonstration
iii. Focused group discussion
iv. Symposium

Q.31. ***Resources include all of the below except:***

i. Money
ii. Material
iii. Manpower
iv. Methodology

Q.32. ***Which type of study is most convenient to undertake to obtain data on health-behavior related aspects of the target population?***

i. Cross-sectional study
ii. Case control study
iii. Cohort study
iv. Ecological study

Q.33. ***Source for assessing health status of the community include all except:***

i. Census office
ii. Registrar of vital events
iii. Civil hospital
iv. Labor office

Q.34. ***Normative needs is:***

i. Needs felt by community
ii. Health needs of community assessed by health workers
iii. Normal day-to-day needs of community
iv. Needs other than health

Q.35. ***Chairperson of health education program should be:***

i. Public health specialist
ii. Influential politician

iii. Superspecialist doctor of concerned topic
iv. Senior teacher

Q.36. ***Target communities are the groups of people who*:**

i. Have the maximum ill-health
ii. Have maximum representation
iii. Are the most influential section of society
iv. Are poor

Q.37. ***Which of the following is an individual health education method?***

i. Lecture
ii. Focused group discussion
iii. Counseling
iv. Newspaper

Q.38. ***Following is/are the type/s of outcome evaluation*:**

i. Concurrent
ii. Terminal
iii. Both
iv. None of the above

Answers

Ans. 1. iv. Housing.

Ans. 2. ii. 16–25.

Ans. 3. iv. 5–10.

Ans. 4. ii. Pareek.

Ans. 5. iii. Housing.

Ans. 6. iii. May be given by the central government.

Ans. 7. i. The date on which one of the family members were vaccinated.

Ans. 8. iii. Summary-sheet.

Ans. 9. iv. Ration card.

Ans. 10. ii. Touch patients appropriately.

Ans. 11. ii. Practice.

Ans. 12. iv. Treatment.

Ans. 13. iv. Accountability.

Ans. 14. i. Social factors in the family.

Ans. 15. i. Total number of family members.

Ans. 16. iv. All of the above.

Ans. 17. i. Village.

Ans. 18. iii. Interaction between family members.

Ans. 19. iv. Support systems.

Ans. 20. ii. Giving money.

Ans. 21. iii. Group discussion.

Ans. 22. iii. Setting an example.

Ans. 23. iv. Demonstration.

Ans. 24. iii. Cultural.

Ans. 25. i. Counseling.

Ans. 26. iv. Defining target communities.

Ans. 27. iv. Defining the premises.

Ans. 28. iv. Resources.

Ans. 29. ii. 2, 1, 4, 3.

Ans. 30. ii. Demonstration.

Ans. 31. iv. Methodology.

Ans. 32. i. Cross-sectional study.

Ans. 33. iv. Labor office.

Ans. 34. ii. Health needs of community assessed by health workers.

Ans. 35. ii. Influential politician.

Ans. 36. i. Have the maximum ill-health.

Ans. 37. iii. Counseling.

Ans. 38. iii. Both.

12 Statistics

Introduction to Biostatistics

Q.1. ***An 85 years old man is rushed to the emergency department by ambulance during an episode of chest pain. The preliminary assessment of the condition of the man is performed by a nurse, who reports that the patients pain seems to be 'severe'. The characterization of pain as 'severe' is:***

i. Dichotomous
ii. Nominal
iii. Quantitative
iv. Qualitative

Q.2. ***If we ask the patient attending OPD to evaluate his pain on a scale of 0 (no pain) to 5 (the worst pain), then this commonly applied scale is a:***

i. Dichotomous
ii. Ratio scale
iii. Continuous
iv. Nominal

Descriptive Statistics: Displaying the Data

Q.3. ***Which of the following is used for representing qualitative data?***

i. Histogram
ii. Polygon
iii. Pie chart
iv. Line chart

Q.4. ***The scatter plot is used to display:***

i. Causality
ii. Correlation
iii. Power
iv. Type II error

Q.5. *5 summary plot consists of quartiles and*:

i. Median
ii. Mode
iii. Mean
iv. Range

Q.6. *The appropriate method of displaying the changes that occur in disease frequency overtime*:

i. Line chart
ii. Bar chart
iii. Histogram
iv. Stem and leaf

Q.7. *Box and whisker plot is also known as*:

i. Magical box
ii. 4 summary plot
iii. 5 summary plot
iv. None of the above

Q.8. *The type of diagram useful to detect linear relationship between two variables is*:

i. Histogram
ii. Line chart
iii. Scatter plot
iv. Bar chart

Q.9. *The following table shows the age distribution of cases of a certain disease reported during a year in a particular state. Which graphical presentation is appropriate to describe this data?*

Age	*Number of cases*
5–14	5
15–24	10
25–34	120
35–44	22
45–54	13
55–64	5

i. Pie chart
ii. Line chart

iii. Histogram
iv. Pictogram

Q.10. ***Which graphical presentation is best to describe the following data?***

Year	*Exports (crores of rupees)*	*Imports (crores of rupees)*
1960–61	610.3	624.65
1961–62	955.39	742.78
1962–63	660.65	578.36
1963–64	585.25	527.98

i. Multiple bar chart
ii. Pie chart
iii. Histogram
iv. Box plot

Q.11. ***Out of the 140 children, 20 lived in owner occupied houses, 70 lived in council houses and 50 lived in private rented accommodation. Type of accommodation is a categorical variable. Appropriate graphical presentation will be:***

i. Line chart
ii. Simple bar chart
iii. Histogram
iv. Frequency polygon

Q.12. ***A study was conducted to assess the awareness of phimosis in young infants and children upto 5 years of age. The awareness level with respect to the family income is as tabulated below. Which graphical presentation is best to describe the following data?***

	< 2000	2000–5000	5000–8000	> 8000
Aware	50	62	77	70
Unaware	50	28	23	30

i. Stem and leaf
ii. Pie chart
iii. Multiple bar chart
iv. Component bar chart

Q.13. ***Following is the frequency distribution of the serum levels of total cholesterol reported in a sample of 71 subjects. Which graphical presentation is best to describe the following data?***

Serum cholesterol level	*Frequency*
<130	2
130–150	7
150–170	18
170–190	20
190–210	15
210–230	7
>230	2
(a) Stem and leaf	(b) Pie (c) Histogram

i. Stem and leaf
ii. Pie
iii. Histogram
iv. Component bar chart

Q.14. ***Information from the sports committee member on representation in different games at the state level by gender is as given below. Which graphical presentation is best to describe the following data?***

Different games	*Females*	*Males*
Long jump	4	6
High jump	2	4
Shot put	9	11
Running	15	10
Swimming	5	4

i. Box plot
ii. Histogram
iii. Multiple bar chart
iv. Pie chart

Q.15. *Which graphical presentation is best to describe the following data?*

Grade of malnutrition	*Frequency*
Normal	60
Grade I	30
Grade II	7
Grade III	2
Grade IV	1

i. Box plot
ii. Component bar chart
iii. Histogram
iv. Pie chart

Summarizing the Data: Measures of Central Tendency and Variability

Q.16. *Which of the statistical average takes into account all the numbers equally?*

i. Mean
ii. Median
iii. Mode
iv. None of the above

Q.17. *Which of the following is a measure of spread?*

i. Variance
ii. Mean
iii. p-value
iv. Mode

Q.18. *Which of the following is a measure of location?*

i. Variance
ii. Mode
iii. p-value
iv. Median

Q.19. *Which among the following is not a measure of variability?*

i. Standard deviation
ii. Range
iii. Median
iv. Coefficient of variation

Q.20. ***For a positively skewed curve which measure of central tendency is largest:***

i. Mean
ii. Mode
iii. Median
iv. All are equal

Q.21. ***Most common value that repeats itself in the data set is:***

i. Mean
ii. Mode
iii. Median
iv. All of the above

Q.22. ***Variance is square of:***

i. p-value
ii. Mean deviation
iii. Standard deviation
iv. Coefficient of variation

Q.23. ***Percentiles divides the data into _____ equal parts:***

i. 100
ii. 50
iii. 10
iv. 25

Q.24. ***10 babies are born in a hospital on same day. All weigh 2.8 kg each: What would be the standard deviation:***

i. 0.28
ii. 1
iii. 2.8
iv. 0

Q.25. ***To compare the variability in two populations we use this measure:***

i. Range
ii. Coefficient of variation
iii. Median
iv. Standard deviation

Introducing Inferential Statistics: Gaussian Distribution and Central Limit Theorem

Q.26. ***Characteristics of normal distribution curve includes all except:***

i. Bell-shaped symmetrical curve

ii. Mean, mode, median coincides
iii. Area under the curve is 1
iv. Mean of all the curves is same

Q.27. ***Area enclosed in normal distribution curve between mean ±2 SD is:***

i. 90%
ii. 95%
iii. 99%
iv. 20%

Q.28. ***Mean of unit normal distribution is:***

i. 1
ii. 0
iii. Unknown
iv. 100

Q.29. ***Variance of unit normal distribution is:***

i. 0
ii. 2
iii. 1
iv. Not known

Q.30. ***Coefficient of kurtosis, β1 measures:***

i. Peakedness of distribution
ii. Skewness of distribution
iii. Spreadness of distribution
iv. All of the above

Q.31. ***All are true regarding normal distribution curve except:***

i. One standard deviation includes 95% of values
ii. Mean, median, mode coincides
iii. Median is mid value
iv. Area under the curve is one

Inferential Statistics: Estimation and Hypothesis Testing

Q.32. ***Standard error of mean shows:***

i. Variation within samples
ii. Variation of sample means from population mean
iii. Both of the above
iv. None of the above

Q.33. ***Type I error is:***

i. Rejecting true null hypothesis
ii. Rejecting false null hypothesis
iii. Accepting true null hypothesis
iv. Accepting false null hypothesis

Q.34. ***Type II error is:***

i. Rejecting true null hypothesis
ii. Rejecting false null hypothesis
iii. Accepting true null hypothesis
iv. Accepting false null hypothesis

Q.35. ***Power is the ability to:***

i. Reject true null hypothesis
ii. Reject false null hypothesis
iii. Accept true null hypothesis
iv. Accept false null hypothesis

Q.36. ***Statistically significant results mean that:***

i. Effect is due to chance
ii. Effect is not due to chance alone
iii. Findings are clinically significant
iv. All of the above

Q.37. ***Type II error and ______ are complimentary:***

i. Type I error
ii. p-value
iii. Power
iv. None of the above

Q.38. ***What is the effect of increasing sample size on power?***

i. It increases
ii. It decreases
iii. It remains same
iv. None of the above

Hypothesis Testing: The Difference between Two Population Proportions

Q.39. ***25 children are chosen randomly from a school playground. Their heights are measured when they first come into school the next morning, and again just before they go home that***

same evening. What statistical test could be used to test the hypothesis that their morning heights are no different from their evening heights?

i. Unpaired t-test
ii. Paired t-test
iii. z-test
iv. Regression

Q.40. ***To label a statistical test definitely significant, the p-value should be:***

i. Less than 0.05
ii. Less than 0.5
iii. Greater than 0.05
iv. Greater than 0.5

Q.41. ***The basic goal of hypothesis testing is:***

i. To confirm the alternative hypothesis
ii. To distinguish between random and meaningful differences in outcome
iii. To establish the value of alpha
iv. To establish the value of beta

Q.42. ***The value of alpha serves as protection against:***

i. False negative results
ii. Inadequate sample size
iii. Type I error
iv. Type II error

Q.43. ***6 volunteers have gone on a cholesterol lowering diet for 6 months. The pretrial and the posttrial changes in the cholesterol levels are as given in the table. The appropriate test of statistical significance for this trial is:***

i. The critical ratio
ii. Odds ratio
iii. Paired t-test
iv. Student's t-test

Q.44. ***In the testing of hypothesis problems, we reject the null hypothesis:***

i. If the test statistic value (calculated) is greater than the table value
ii. If the test statistic value (calculated) is smaller than the table value

iii. If the test statistic value (calculated) is equal to the table value
iv. None of the above

Q.45. ***In comparing the difference between two population means, if value of p is 0.31. Then correct interpretation is:***

i. There is a significant difference between population means
ii. There is no significant difference between population means
iii. None of the above
iv. All of the above

Q.46. ***In a small sample survey on 7 male and 10 female students, the mean cholesterol levels were found to be 250 mg% and 260 mg% respectively. Which one of the following statistical tests is appropriate to find significance of the difference in this case:***

i. Chi-square test
ii. Unpaired t-test
iii. Paired t-test
iv. z-test

Q.47. ***The statistical test used to analyze the difference between the mean values of hemoglobin of two independent samples (of 100 school children in each sample) drawn from normally distributed populations is:***

i. Paired t-test
ii. Unpaired t-test
iii. Chi-square test
iv. z-test

Q.48. ***The minimum power of a study should be:***

i. 70%
ii. 80%
iii. 90%
iv. None of the above

Q.49. ***Hb of 10 people was measured before and after giving them iron tablets for 1 month. Statistical test which can be used to measure the effect of iron on Hb is:***

i. Paired t-test
ii. Unpaired t-test

iii. Sign test
iv. Chi-square test

Q.50. ***In hypothesis testing between two population means null hypothesis is:***

i. $\mu 1 = \mu 2$
ii. $\mu 1 = 0$
iii. $\mu 1 = \mu 2 = 0$
iv. $\mu 1 \neq \mu 2$

Q.51. ***Paired t-test is used in all the following condition except:***

i. When only one sample gives two sets of readings (before and after readings)
ii. When two different samples are similar to each (paired match)
iii. When two different samples are similar to each (frequency match)
iv. Independent samples are considered

Q.52. ***If numerical ordinal data for paired samples is used then the statistical test used is:***

i. Sign test
ii. Wilcoxon sign test
iii. Paired t-test
iv. Chi-square test

Q.53. ***Researcher's interest is to see whether the two samples that he/she has drawn, differ significantly from each other as regards the "mean" of a particular variable of interest the statistical procedure used is:***

i. Hypothesis testing of difference between two means
ii. Hypothesis testing of single mean
iii. Chi-square test
iv. All of the above

Q.54. ***While testing a hypolipidemic drug, serum lipids levels were tested both before and after its use. Which test is best suited for the statistical analysis of the results?***

i. Paired t-test
ii. Unpaired t-test
iii. Chi-square test
iv. All of the above

Chi-square Test

Q.55. ***In a study to determine relationship between presence of IHD and smoking, the appropriate statistical test is:***

i. z-test
ii. Paired t-test
iii. Chi-square test
iv. None of the above

Q.56. ***Which of the following is nonparametric test?***

i. z-test
ii. t-test
iii. Chi-square test
iv. None of the above

Q.57. ***Under the null hypothesis the test statistic follows a chi-square distribution with ____________ degrees of freedom:***

i. (r–1) × (c–1)
ii. r × c
iii. n
iv. n–1

Q.58. ***All are application of chi-square test except:***

i. χ^2 test for independence
ii. χ^2 test for goodness of fit
iii. χ^2 test for homogeneity
iv. χ^2 test for heterogenicity

Q.59. ***The number of degrees of freedom in a table of (4*4) in chi-square test is:***

i. 16
ii. 8
iii. 9
iv. 1

Confidence Interval

Q.60. ***95% of confidence limits exist between:***

i. +1SD
ii. + 2SD
iii. + 3SD
iv. + 4SD

Q.61. ***Wider the range of confidence interval:***

i. More is the precision of estimate
ii. Precision does not get affected by it
iii. Less is the precision of estimate
iv. None of the above

Q.62. ***Hypothesized null value for confidence interval of relative risk:***

i. 0
ii. 1
iii. 2
iv. 5

Q.63. ***If confidence interval includes null value then the results are:***

i. Statistically not significant
ii. Statistically significant
iii. Clinically significant
iv. None of the above

Q.64. ***95% confidence interval means that we are:***

i. 5% error in our estimation of population parameter
ii. 95% close to the estimation of population parameter
iii. 95% confident that parameter will lie in this range
iv. None of the above

Sampling Methods

Q.65. ***The list of each and every individual in the population is called as:***

i. Sampling frame
ii. Sampling error
iii. Sampling ratio
iv. Sampling procedure

Q.66. ***All is true about simple random sample sampling except:***

i. Impractical if N is very large
ii. Minority subgroups are adequately represented
iii. Every member has an equal chance of being included
iv. Population estimate is easy to calculate

Q.67. ***Probability samplings are all except:***

i. Simple random sampling
ii. Systematic random sampling
iii. Cluster sampling
iv. Quota sampling

Q.68. ***In simple random sampling if the subject is replaced back in the population it is termed as:***

i. Simple random sampling with replacement
ii. Simple random sampling without replacement
iii. Systematic sampling
iv. None of the above

Q.69. ***Requirements of a sample is that it should be:***

i. Representative
ii. Adequate
iii. None of the above
iv. Both (i) and (ii)

Simple Correlation and Regression

Q.70. ***The scatter plot is used to display:***

i. Causality
ii. Correlation
iii. Power
iv. Type II error

Q.71. ***The correct statistical procedure for studying the association between an exposure and an outcome variable when both of them are measured on a continuous scale is:***

i. Chi-square test
ii. Pearson's correlation coefficient
iii. ANOVA
iv. t-test

Q.72. ***In regression equation Y = a + bx, b represents:***

i. Intercept on Y-axis
ii. Slope of the line
iii. Intercept on X-axis
iv. None of the above

Q.73. ***If correlation coefficient r = 0 it implies:***

i. Perfect positive linear relationship
ii. Perfect negative linear relationship
iii. No linear relationship
iv. None of the above

Q.74. ***When the variables are not normally distributed but are ranked in order then the appropriate correlation measure is:***

i. Spearman rank correlation coefficients
ii. Karl Pearson product moment correlation
iii. Wilcoxon sign test
iv. None of the above

Standardization of Rates

Q.75. ***All are true regarding direct standardization except:***

i. Age specific death rate is required for comparison
ii. Age composition of the standard population is required
iii. Vital statistics are required
iv. Without knowledge of the age composition, the two populations can be compared

Q.76. ***Which method is used for controlling the effect of potential confounders during the analysis stage of large scale field research work?***

i. Standardization
ii. Matching
iii. Restriction
iv. All of the above

Q.77. ***Which statement is true:***

i. Standardized mortality rate are actual rate
ii. For indirect standardization age specific mortality rate are required
iii. Standardized mortality rate are imaginary
iv. Standardization is done in planning stage

Q.78. ***Standardized mortality ratio is calculated in:***

i. Indirect standardization
ii. Direct standardization

iii. Both
iv. None

Q.79. ***Direct standardization is also known as:***

i. Changing base method
ii. Fixed base method
iii. Hanging base method
iv. None of the above

Advanced Statistical Procedures

A. NONPARAMETRIC TEST:

Q.80. ***An obstetrician takes two groups of expectant ladies from her ANC-one group having anemia while the other did not have anemia. She follows them till delivery and notes the APGAR score of baby, to see if anemia in pregnancy was associated with a lower APGAR score in newborn. The correct statistical procedure in this study would be:***

i. t-test
ii. Mann-Whitney test
iii. Odds ratio
iv. Correlation coefficient

Q.81. ***All of the following are nonparametric test except:***

i. Mann-Whitney test
ii. Wilcoxon sign test
iii. Chi-square test
iv. t-test

Q.82. ***All of the following are correct except:***

i. Nonparametric test are stronger than parametric test
ii. Nonparametric test are also known as distribution free test
iii. Chi-square is a nonparametric test
iv. None of the above

Q.83. ***For comparing the median of two population statistical test used is:***

i. z-test
ii. t-test
iii. Mann-Whitney test
iv. All of the above

Q.84. ***Wilcoxan signed rank test takes into account:***

i. Direction of differences
ii. Magnitude of differences
iii. Both
iv. None of the above

B. ANOVA:

Q.85. ***When more than two treatment groups are present and you wish to test whether the groups differ significantly with respect to a parameter which statistical method would be applied?***

i. ANCOVA
ii. ANOVA
iii. Logistic regression method
iv. Multivariate regression

Q.86. ***The correct technique to compare difference in three or more groups when homogeneity condition fails is:***

i. z-test
ii. t-test
iii. ANOVA
iv. Kruskal Wallis test

Q.87. ***Assumption that variance in all the group is same, is tested by:***

i. Wilcoxan sign test
ii. Bartlett's test
iii. Bonferroni's procedure
iv. Schaffe's method

Q.88. ***All of the following are multiple comparison test except:***

i. Bonferroni's procedure
ii. Schaffe's method
iii. Newman-Keul's procedure
iv. Wilcoxan sign test

Q.89. ***Pairwise comparison between the groups or treatments when F ratio is significant is carried using:***

i. Paired t-test
ii. Unpaired t-test
iii. Bonferroni's test
iv. Duncan's test

C. CONTROL OF CONFOUNDING, LINEAR TREND AND PAIRED DATA ANALYSIS:

Q.90. ***When data is dichotomous and are matched paired, what is the correct statistical test?***

i. Paired t-test
ii. Mantel-Haenszel chi-square test
iii. McNemar's chi-square test
iv. Chi-square test for linear trend

Q.91. ***All are true of confounder variable except*:**

i. It is related to exposure
ii. It is related to outcome
iii. It is indirect chain of causation from exposure to outcome
iv. It is differentially distributed

Q.92. ***If stratum odds ratios are different from each other it means*:**

i. Confounding is present
ii. Effect modification is there
iii. No effect
iv. All of the above

Q.93. ***If stratum odds ratios are different from crude ratio then*:**

i. Confounding is present
ii. Effect modification is there
iii. No effect
iv. All of the above

Q.94. ***When the researcher is dealing with qualitative ordinal variables the analysis is done by*:**

i. Analyzing proportion in various categories
ii. Chi-square for linear trend
iii. McNemar's chi-square test
iv. Sign test

Answers

Ans. 1. iv. Qualitative.

Ans. 2. ii. Ratio scale.

Ans. 3. iii. Pie chart.

Ans. 4. ii. Correlation.

Ans. 5. i. Median.

Ans. 6. i. Line chart.

Ans. 7. iii. 5 summary plot.

Ans. 8. iii. Scatter plot.

Ans. 9. iii. Histogram.

Ans. 10. i. Multiple bar chart.

Ans. 11. ii. Simple bar chart.

Ans. 12. iv. Component bar chart.

Ans. 13. iii. Histogram.

Ans. 14. iii. Multiple bar chart.

Ans. 15. iv. Pie chart.

Ans. 16. i. Mean.

Ans. 17. i. Variance.

Ans. 18. iv. Median.

Ans. 19. iii. Median.

Ans. 20. i. Mean.

Ans. 21. ii. Mode.

Ans. 22. iii. Standard deviation.

Ans. 23. i. 100.

Ans. 24. iv. 0.

Ans. 25. ii. Coefficient of variation.

Ans. 26. iv. Mean of all the curves is same.

Ans. 27. ii. 95%.

Ans. 28. ii. 0.

Ans. 29. iii. 1.

Ans. 30. i. Peakedness of distribution.

Ans. 31. i. One standard deviation includes 95% of values.

Ans. 32. ii. Variation of sample means from population mean.

Ans. 33. i. Rejecting true null hypothesis.

Ans. 34. iv. Accepting false null hypothesis.

Ans. 35. ii. Reject false null hypothesis.

Ans. 36. ii. Effect is not due to chance alone.

Ans. 37. iii. Power.

Ans. 38. i. It increases.

Ans. 39. ii. Paired t-test.

Ans. 40. i. Less than 0.05.

Ans. 41. ii. To distinguish between random and meaningful differences in outcome.

Ans. 42. iii. Type I error.

Ans. 43. iii. Paired t-test.

Ans. 44. i. If the test statistic value (calculated) is greater than the table value.

Ans. 45. ii. There is no significant difference between population means.

Ans. 46. ii. Unpaired t-test.

Ans. 47. iv. z-test.

Ans. 48. ii. 80%.

Ans. 49. i. Paired t-test.

Ans. 50. i. $\mu 1 = \mu 2$.

Ans. 51. iii. When two different samples are similar to each (frequency match).

Ans. 52. ii. Wilcoxon sign test.

Ans. 53. i. Hypothesis testing of difference between two means.

Ans. 54. i. Paired t-test.

Ans. 55. iii. Chi-square test.

Ans. 56. iii. Chi-square test.

Ans. 57. i. $(r-1) \times (c-1)$.

Ans. 58. iv. χ^2 test for heterogenicity.

Ans. 59. iii. 9.

Ans. 60. ii. + 2SD.

Ans. 61. iii. Less is the precision of estimate.

Ans. 62. ii. 1.

Ans. 63. i. Statistically not significant.

Ans. 64. i. 5% error in our estimation of population parameter.

Ans. 65. i. Sampling frame.

Ans. 66. ii. Minority subgroups are adequately represented.

Ans. 67. iv. Quota sampling.

Ans. 68. i. Simple random sampling with replacement.

Ans. 69. iv. Both (i) and (ii).

Ans. 70. ii. Correlation.

Ans. 71. ii. Pearson's correlation coefficient.

Ans. 72. ii. Slope of the line.

Ans. 73. iii. No linear relationship.

Ans. 74. i. Spearman rank correlation coefficients.

Ans. 75. iv. Without knowledge of the age composition, the two populations can be compared.

Ans. 76. i. Standardization.

Ans. 77. iii. Standardized mortality rate are imaginary.

Ans. 78. i. Indirect standardization.

Ans. 79. ii. Fixed base method.

Ans. 80. ii. Mann-Whitney test.

Ans. 81. iv. t-test.

Ans. 82. i. Nonparametric test are stronger than parametric test.

Ans. 83. iii. Mann-Whitney test.

Ans. 84. iii. Both.

Ans. 85. ii. ANOVA.

Ans. 86. iv. Kruskal Wallis test.

Ans. 87. ii. Bartlett's test.

Ans. 88. iv. Wilcoxan sign test.

Ans. 89. iii. Bonferroni's test.

Ans. 90. iii. McNemar's chi-square test.

Ans. 91. iii. It is indirect chain of causation from exposure to outcome.

Ans. 92. ii. Effect modification is there.

Ans. 93. i. Confounding is present.

Ans. 94. ii. Chi-square for linear trend.

Appendix I

Health Benefits of Various Fruits

Amazing Benefits of Bananas

Energy
Bananas supply proper carbohydrates necessary to replace the muscle glycogen (muscle sugar) used

Bowel health
Bananas are high in soluble fiber which helps to stop constipation and restore, and to maintain regular bowel function

Increase happiness
Bananas release a mood regulating substance called tryptophan which is converted to serotonin in the brain and thus elevates mood and makes us happier!

Potassium
High in potassium, bananas help the body's circulatory system deliver oxygen to the brain, helping maintain regular heartbeat and proper water balance in

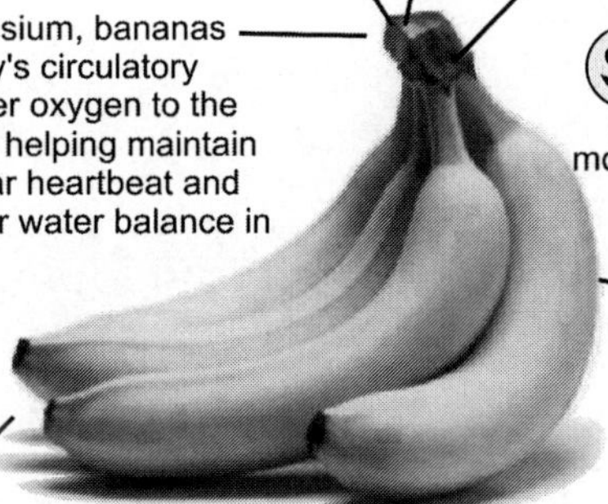

Help smokers quit
Bananas contain B vitamins and other minerals that lessen the effects of nicotine withdrawal both physically and psychologically

PMS
Bananas contain vitamin B_6. This vitamin regulates blood glucose levels and helps us in times of stress and helps to suppress cranky moods

Brain power
Potassium-packed fruit helps learning because it makes the pupils more alert. Students find that they have more brain power and do better on exams when they eat bananas at breakfast and lunch

Iron
Bananas are rich in iron too and can help individuals with anemia. Iron rich foods, such as bananas help stimulate production of hemoglobin in the blood

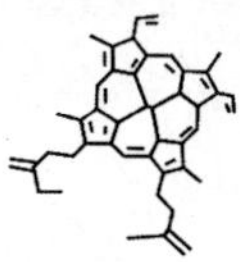

Beets are excellent cancer fighters

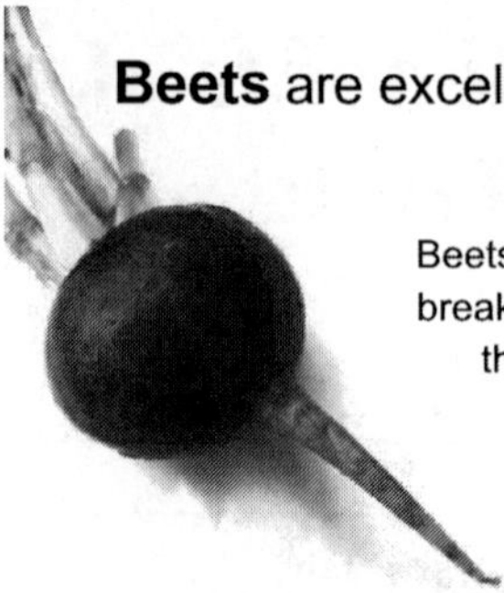

Beets are strongly effective in breaking up tumors mainly by their excellent amount of betacyanin.

Betacyanin is the main ingredient that causes red beet its purple reddish color.

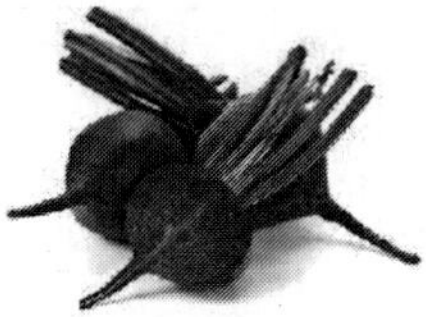

Ancient Chinese bean prevents hospital death

Sepsis is a life-threatening complication of an infection or injury.

It triggers an overpowering inflammatory response throughout the body that can lead to shock, organ failure, and possible death. Sepsis inflicts irreversible damage on vital organs such as the liver, heart, lungs, kidneys and brain.

Sepsis affects 750,000 Americans every year and 28–50% of them die.

In a promising study researchers have found that mung bean extract increases survival rate of sepsis from 29–70%!

In addition mung beans protect against heart disease.

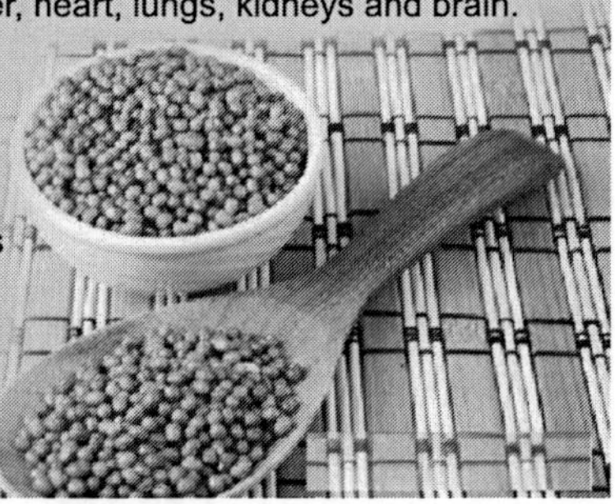

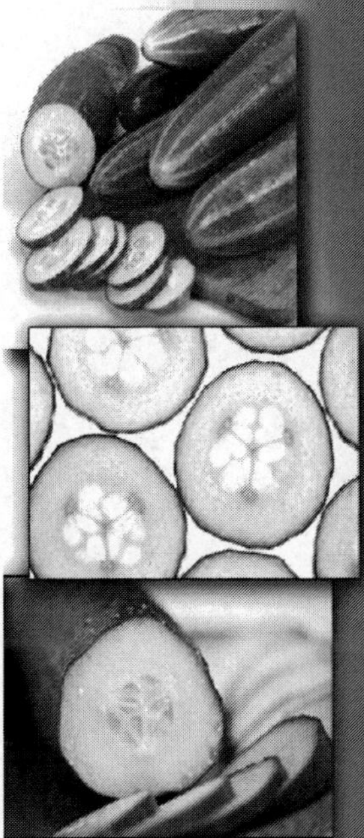

Top health benefits of cucumber

*Keep body hydrated-cucumber has 96% water content that is more nutritious than regular water

*Skin care

The high water content, vitamins A, B and C, and the presence of certain minerals like magnesium, potassium, and silica make cucumbers an essential part of skin care

*Control blood pressure

Cucumber juice contains a lot of potassium, magnesium and fiber that work effectively for regulating blood pressure

*Aid digestion

Digestive disorders like acidity, heartburn, gastritis and even ulcers can be cured by the daily consumption of fresh cucumber juice

*Relieve gout and arthritis pain

Cucumber is rich in vitamin A, B_1, B_6, C and D, folate, calcium, magnesium and potassium, when mixed with carrot juice, they can relieve gout and arthritis pain by lowering the uric acid levels

*Aid in weight loss

Due to its low calorie and high water content, cucumber is an ideal diet for people who looking for weight loss.

Crazy for coconut

Top 10 reasons I love cocount oil

1. Rich in nutrients, fiber, vitamins and minerals.
2. Naturally antiviral, antimicrobial, antiprotozoal and antifungal, it kills the bad stuff inside and outside your body.
3. Boosts energy, endurance, thyroid function and metabolism to prevent obesity and assist in weight loss.
4. Reduces health risk of diabetes by improving insulin and blood glucose functions.
5. Protects against osteoporosis by improving calcium and magnesium absorption, builds strong bones and teeth.
6. Protects the body against various forms of cancer.
7. Supports healing and repair of skin and protects from free-radicals that promote aging.
8. The lauric acid in coconut oil works as a natural underarm deodorant by killing odor causing bacteria.
9. Softens skin, conditions hair, prevents wrinkles, sags and age spots, controls dandruff.
10. Has no harmful side effects.

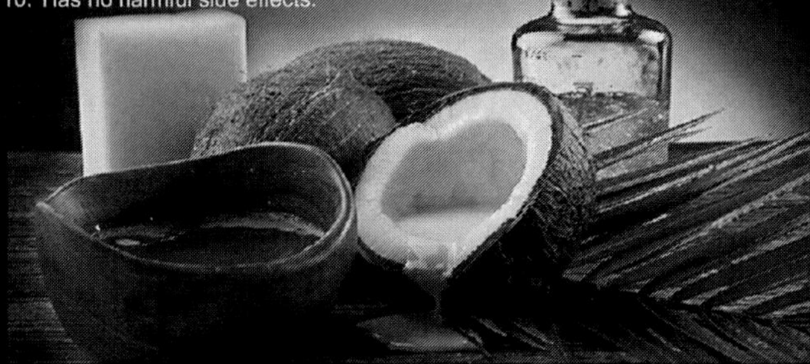

Health benefits of cinnamon

1. Cinnamon has antifungal, antibacterial and antiparasitic properties
2. Cinnamon has anti-inflammatory properties.
3. Cinnamon is an excellent source of manganese, dietary fiber, iron and calcium.

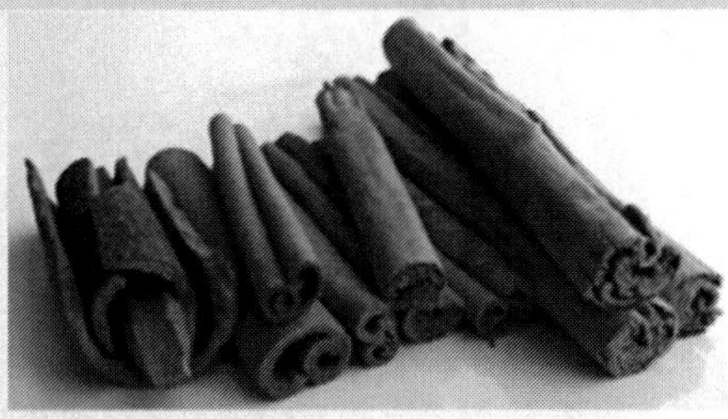

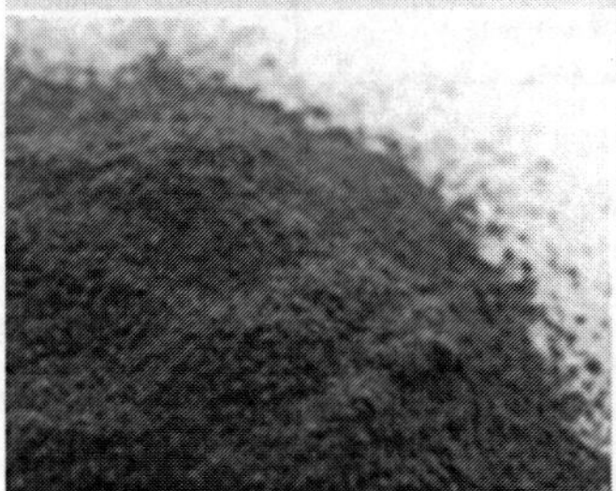

4. Cinnamon boosts the activity of the brain and hence acts as a good brain tonic. It helps in removing nervous tension and memory loss.
5. Cinnamon has also been found useful for women's health as it helps in providing relief from menstrual cramping and other feminine discomforts.
6. When added to food, it prevents bacterial growth and food spoilage, making it a natural food preservative.
7. Cinnamon helps in removing blood impurities. Therefore, it is often recommended for pimples.

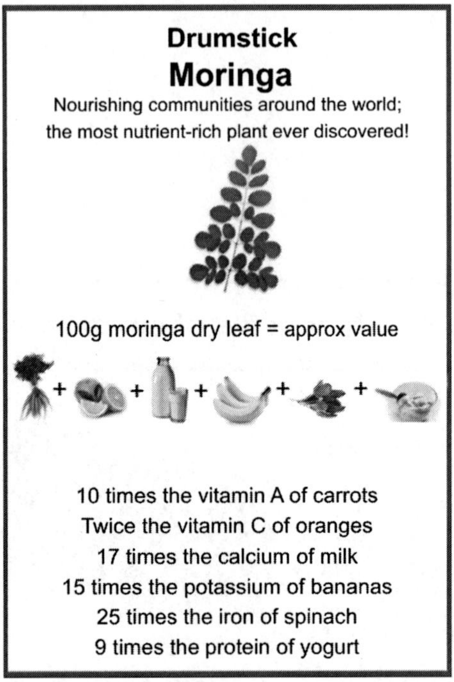
Drumstick
Moringa
Nourishing communities around the world;
the most nutrient-rich plant ever discovered!
100g moringa dry leaf = approx value
+ + + + +
10 times the vitamin A of carrots
Twice the vitamin C of oranges
17 times the calcium of milk
15 times the potassium of bananas
25 times the iron of spinach
9 times the protein of yogurt

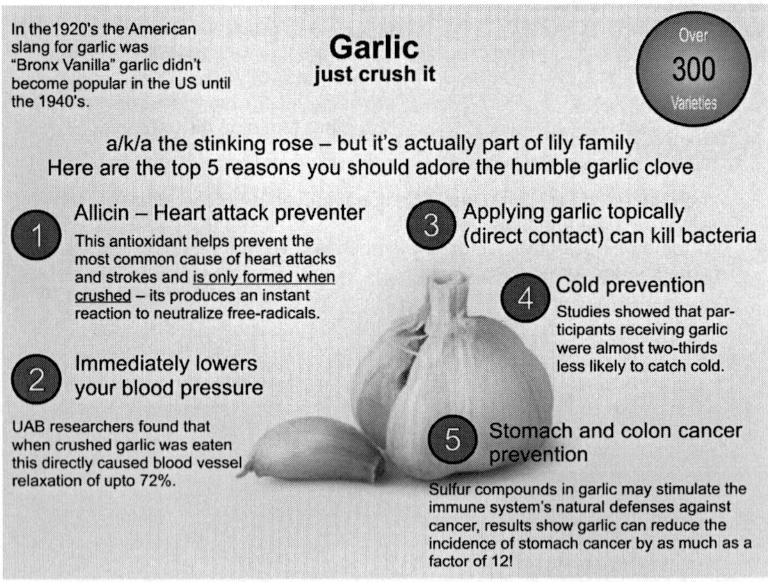
In the1920's the American slang for garlic was "Bronx Vanilla" garlic didn't become popular in the US until the 1940's.
Garlic
just crush it
Over
300
Varieties
a/k/a the stinking rose – but it's actually part of lily family
Here are the top 5 reasons you should adore the humble garlic clove
1
Allicin – Heart attack preventer
This antioxidant helps prevent the most common cause of heart attacks and strokes and is only formed when crushed – its produces an instant reaction to neutralize free-radicals.
2
Immediately lowers your blood pressure
UAB researchers found that when crushed garlic was eaten this directly caused blood vessel relaxation of upto 72%.
3
Applying garlic topically (direct contact) can kill bacteria
4
Cold prevention
Studies showed that participants receiving garlic were almost two-thirds less likely to catch cold.
5
Stomach and colon cancer prevention
Sulfur compounds in garlic may stimulate the immune system's natural defenses against cancer, results show garlic can reduce the incidence of stomach cancer by as much as a factor of 12!

Balance your blood sugar with green tea

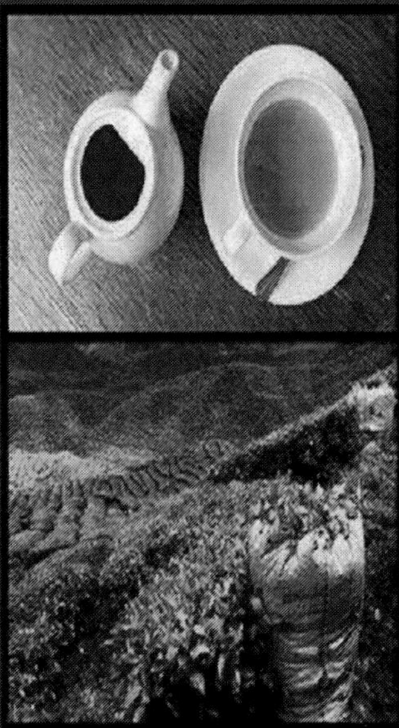

Did you know...that drinking green tea with starchy food may lower blood sugar spikes?

What is it about green tea?

Green tea helps prevent and treat diabetes by increasing insulin activity by more than 15 fold.

NB: Consume in moderation recommended only 2 nos per day.

Animal studies have shown that substances in green tea called polysaccharides mimic insulin and lower blood sugar levels by restricting the amount of glucose the liver produces.

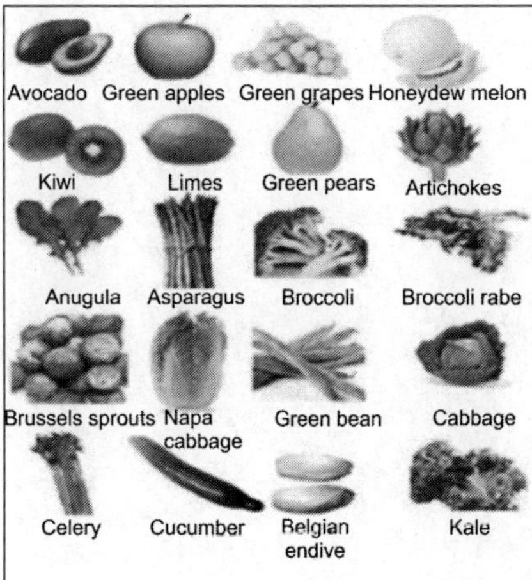

Health benefits of greens

Green vegetables contain chlorophyll, fiber, lutein, zeaxanthin, calcium, folate, vitamin C, calcium, and beta-carotene. The nutrients found in these vegetables reduce cancer risks, lower blood pressure and LDL cholesterol levels. They normalize digestion time, support retinal health and vision. They also fight against harmful free-radicals and boost immune system activity.

Nourish your heart with Omega-3

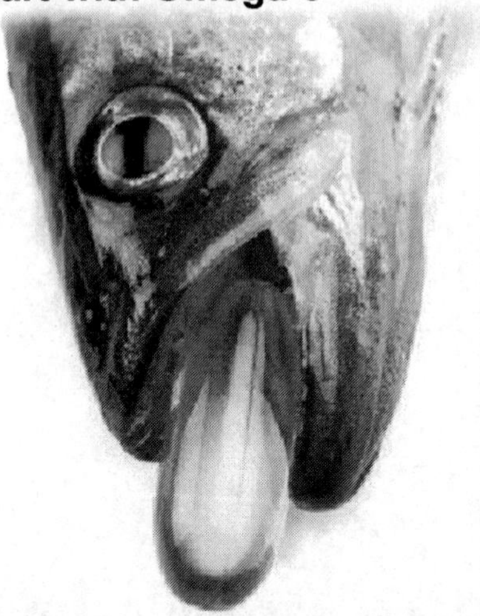

Did you know...that Omega-3s dramatically lower your risk of heart disease...can help prevent atherosclerosis, hypertension and high cholesterol?

Omega-3s have been proven to strengthen your overall heart health. After all, heart disease is the number one killer disease.

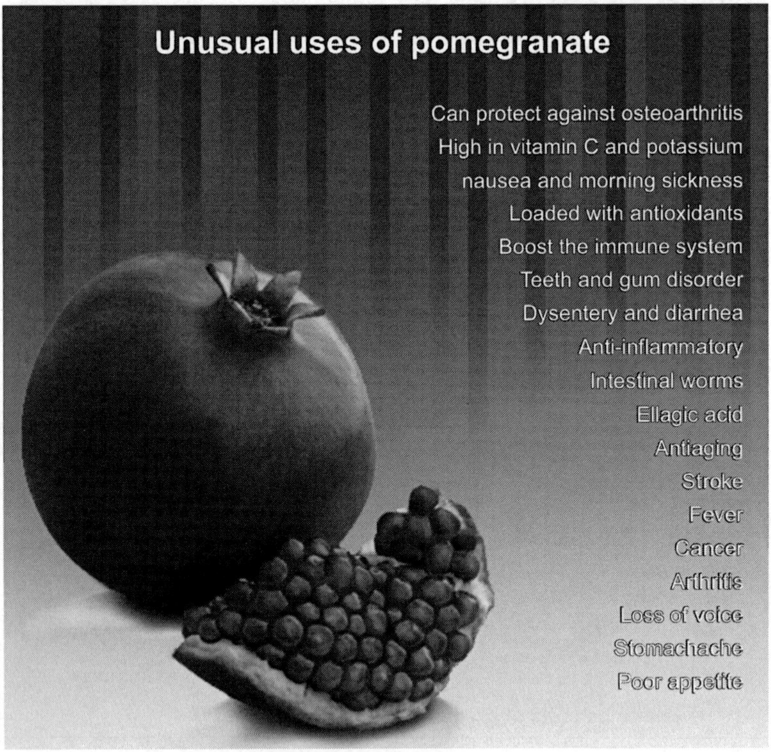
Unusual uses of pomegranate
Can protect against osteoarthritis
High in vitamin C and potassium
nausea and morning sickness
Loaded with antioxidants
Boost the immune system
Teeth and gum disorder
Dysentery and diarrhea
Anti-inflammatory
Intestinal worms
Ellagic acid
Antiaging
Stroke
Fever
Cancer
Arthritis
Loss of voice
Stomachache
Poor appetite

Take a *green* step...

Pumpkin seeds

- Sleep aid
- Heart healer
- Blood builder

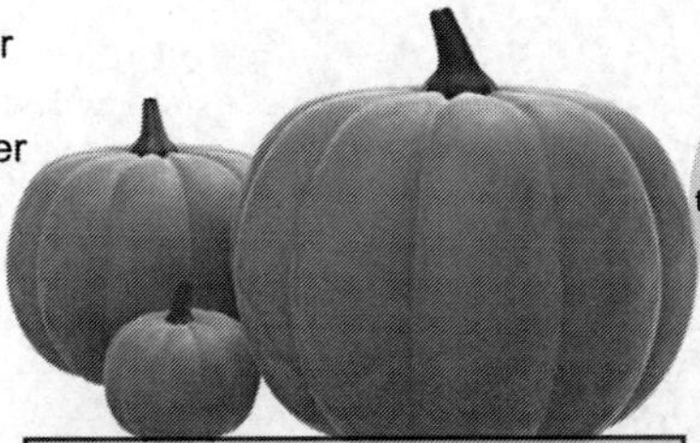

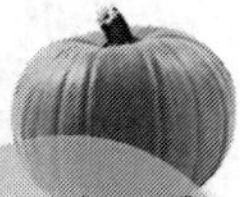

Did you know?
Pumpkin seeds are a sleep aid! They contain the amino acid tryptophan which converts to serotonin, giving you a great nights sleep. Sweet dreams!

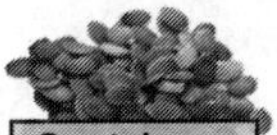

Contains...
vitamin C
vitamin A
magnesium
potassium
zinc
and
fiber

The health benefits of pumpkins are in the seeds.

Pumpkin seeds are rich in easily digestable proteins which maintain healthy blood sugar. Healthy blood sugar is key in weight loss.They are high in magnesium which is great for the heart, and is also a natural relaxant.

Men's health
Pumpkin seeds are high in zinc, which is very good for the prostate. Great snack for men!

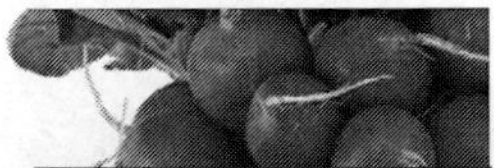

Health benefits of radish

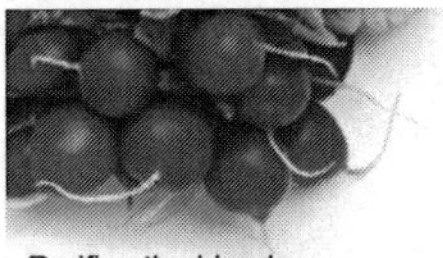

Purifies the blood
facilitates digestion
increases urine production
inhibits kidney infection
anti-inflammatory
rich in vitamin-C, folic acid and anthocyanins
effective for skin disorders
anticongestive, good mouth and breath freshener
effective in fighting oral cancer, colon, kidney and cancers

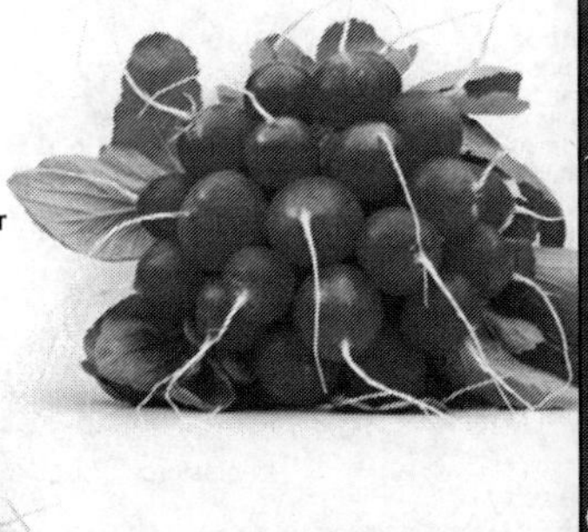

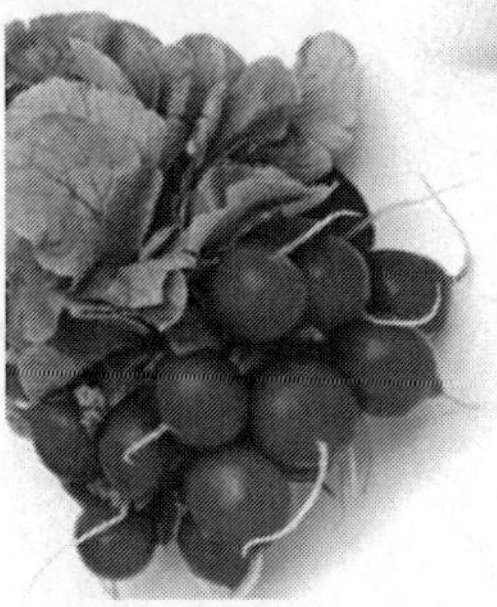

Useful in treatment of leukoderma
helps to regulate blood pressure
beneficial for gallbladder and liver functions remove excess bilirubin from the blood low in calories, cholesterol and fat
helps with constipation and piles natural diuretic
helps with fever

Carrot, orange and radish salad

4 carrots
6 radishes
1 handful fresh mint leaves
1 handful fresh cilantro leaves
2 navel oranges
1/2 teaspoon ground cinnamon
1/2 teaspoon honey
1/2 lemon, juiced
1 teaspoon orange flower water
kosher salt

Slice carrots and radishes as thinly as possible and add to a large bowl. Add mint and cilantro. Remove the peel and pith from the oranges. Working over a bowl to catch the juice, cut between the membranes to remove the orange segments, add to carrots. Squeeze the membrane to extract the rest of the juice and add the cinnamon, sugar (or honey), lemon juice, orange flower water and salt, to taste. Mix to dissolve sugar and salt. Pour over the carrot mixture and gently toss to cost. Allow it to sit for 1–2 hours to help flavors to blend.

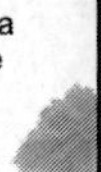

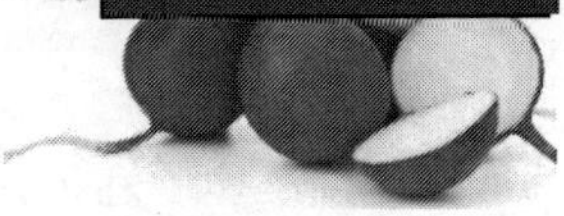

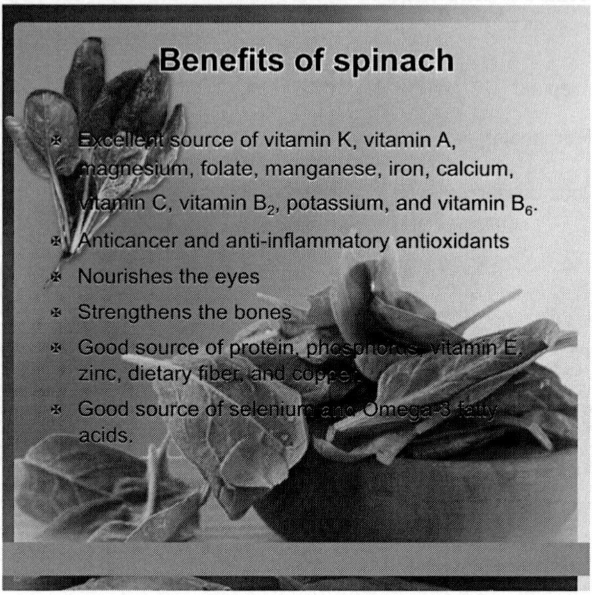
Benefits of spinach
Excellent source of vitamin K, vitamin A, magnesium, folate, manganese, iron, calcium, vitamin C, vitamin B_2, potassium, and vitamin B_6.
Anticancer and anti-inflammatory antioxidants
Nourishes the eyes
Strengthens the bones
Good source of protein, phosphorus, vitamin E, zinc, dietary fiber, and copper.
Good source of selenium and Omega-3 fatty acids.

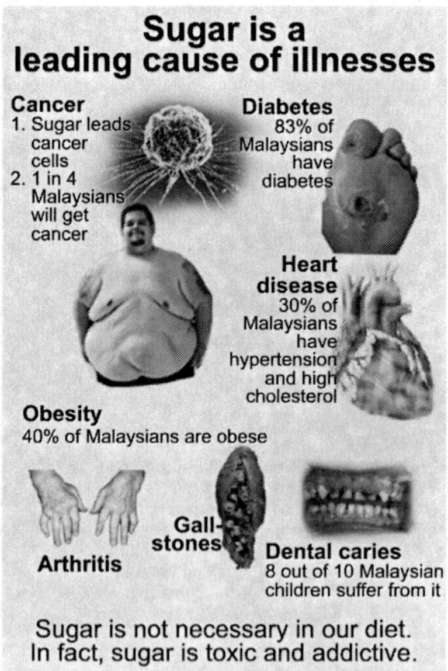
Sugar is a leading cause of illnesses
Cancer
1. Sugar leads cancer cells
2. 1 in 4 Malaysians will get cancer
Diabetes
83% of Malaysians have diabetes
Heart disease
30% of Malaysians have hypertension and high cholesterol
Obesity
40% of Malaysians are obese
Arthritis
Gall-stones
Dental caries
8 out of 10 Malaysian children suffer from it
Sugar is not necessary in our diet.
In fact, sugar is toxic and addictive.

Walnuts

powerful enough to be a cancer drug?

How walnuts may prevent breast cancer

Omega-3 is found in walnuts also inhibits an anti-inflammatory enzyme that advances breast cancer, and activates two genes—BRCA1 and BRCA2 (breast cancer genes 1 and 2)—that helps to prevent cancer development.

7 It only takes 7 walnuts a day to get all the health benefits! 7

In yet another attempt to suppress our health freedom, the (US FDA) issued a warning to walnut producers stating that their claims for the health-promoting qualities of walnuts–which are all substantiated have moved walnuts from a food to a drug!

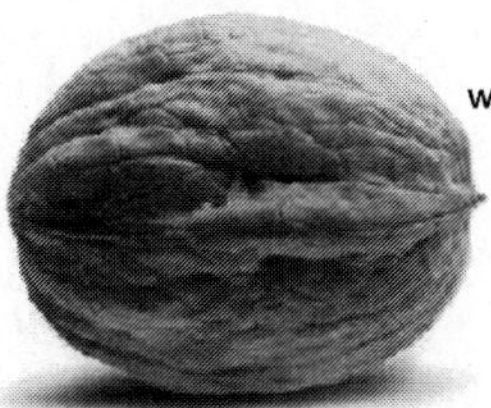

Packed with essential Omega–3

- Reduces blood pressure
- Lowers cholesterol
- Relieves IBS
- Soothes arthritis

Cancer fighting warriors

The highly potent phytonutrient quinone juglone, abundant in walnuts, destroys cancer and precancerous cells while leaving healthy tissue intact.

The Romans called walnuts "Jupiter's royal acorn" and were reserved for royalty.

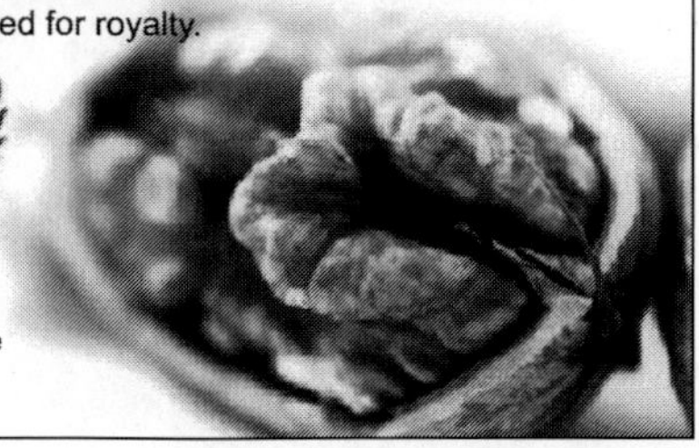

Eat the skin, over 90% of the nutrients are found in the skin.

Appendix II

Certain Signs and Symptoms

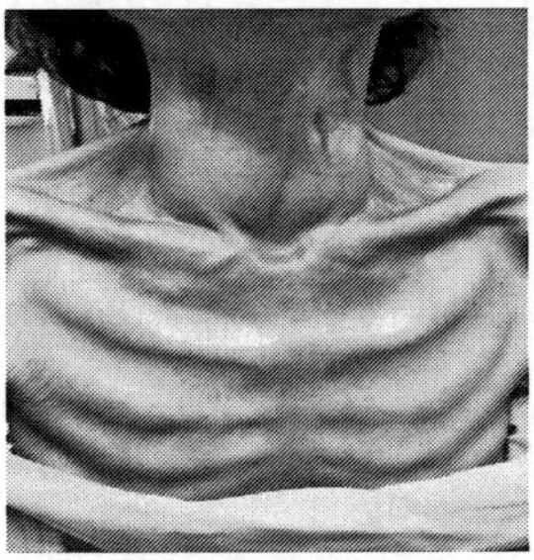

Explanation: Graves' disease

The patient is diaphoretic, cachectic, and has a diffusely enlarged thyroid. These features are most consistent with Graves' disease. The patient had substantial improvement following treatment with methimazole.

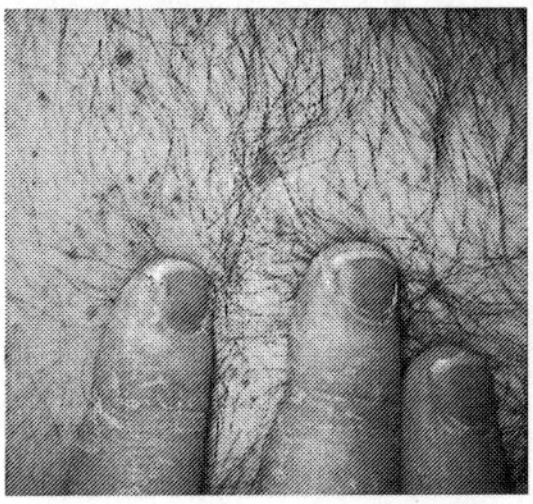

Explanation: Endocarditis

Typical subungual "splinter" hemorrhage and numerous petechiae on the skin of the abdomen are seen in a patient with staphylococcal endocarditis.

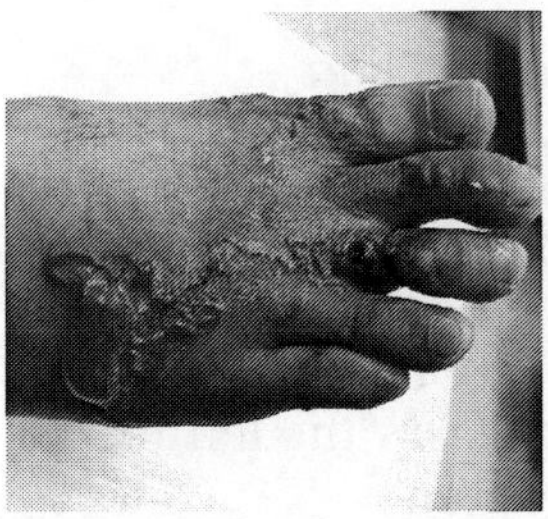

Explanation: Cutaneous larva migrans

The serpiginous, erythematous raised tracts with bulla formation are clinically diagnostic of cutaneous larva migrans. This is the infection of the skin with the hookworm parasite of dogs and cats, *Ancylostoma braziliense.* Eggs in animal feces hatch and mature in the soil and are able to invade human skin. The larva cannot complete it's lifecycle in a human host and it meanders in the skin before dieing.

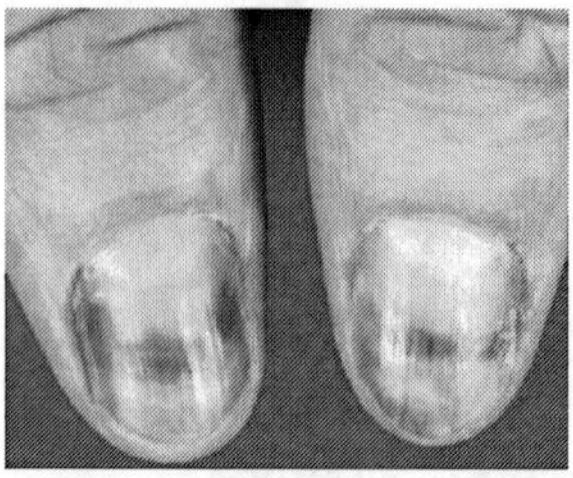

Explanation

Green nails, a form of chromonychia, may be caused by bacterial infection with *P. aeruginosa*. This syndrome is typically seen in patients with nail disease such as onycholysis, onychotillomania, or paronychia, particularly in those whose abnormal nails have been exposed to moist environments. The green color is caused by the fluorescent siderophore pyoverdin, produced by *P. aeruginosa*.

After 2 weeks of treatment with topical nadifloxacin, the nail color returned to normal.

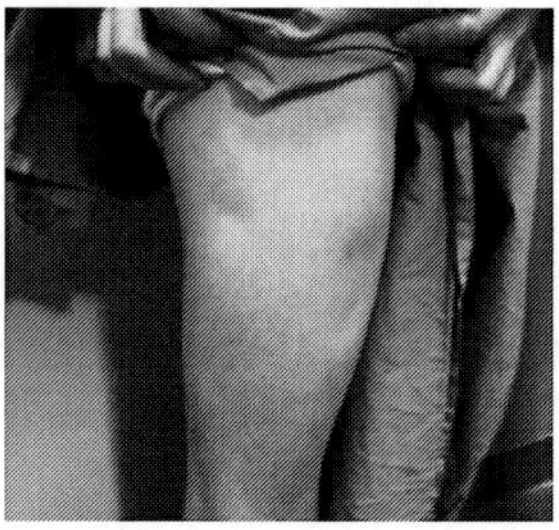

Explanation: Lipoatrophy

Depressed areas of skin at the sites typically used for insulin injection are most consistent with injection-site lipoatrophy. It is associated with all types of insulin and may lead to erratic insulin absorption.

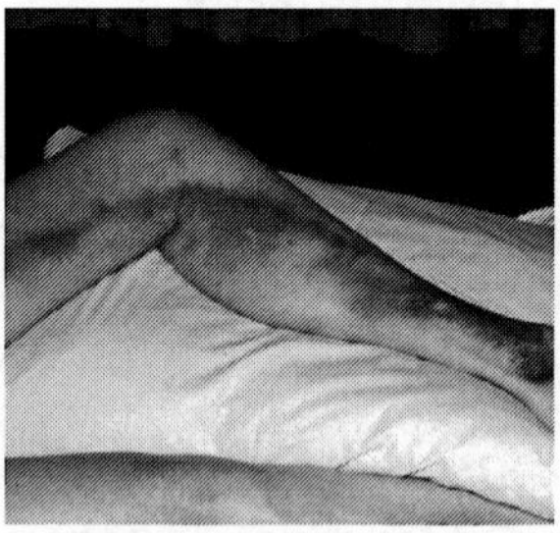

Explanation: Superficial thrombophlebitis

The patient had erythema and tenderness on the medial aspect of the left knee. A palpable, rope-like cord was present from the left medial malleolus to the groin.

Duplex Doppler ultrasonography revealed thrombosis of the greater saphenous vein, with no extension into the deep venous system, consistent with superficial thrombophlebitis.

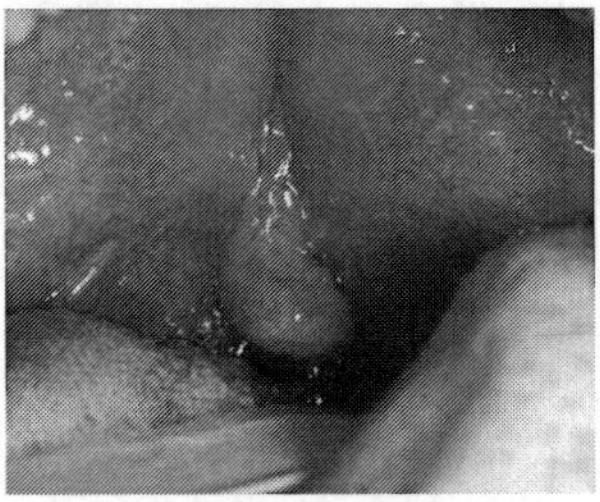

Explanation: Bilateral peritonsillar abscesses

Bilateral swelling of the soft palate is visible with a midline uvula pushed anteriorly. This is most consistent with a diagnosis of bilateral peritonsillar abscesses. Quinsy is a complication of acute tonsillitis, usually due to streptococcal infection. It is a collection of pus arising outside the capsule of the tonsil in close relationship to its upper pole.

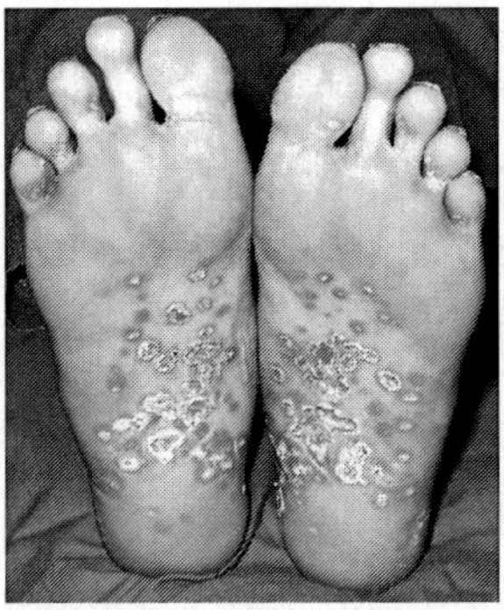

Explanation: Keratoderma blennorrhagicum

These vesiculopustular waxy lesions are most consistent with keratoderma blennorrhagicum. This finding should prompt diagnostic testing for sexually transmitted or gastrointestinal pathogens.

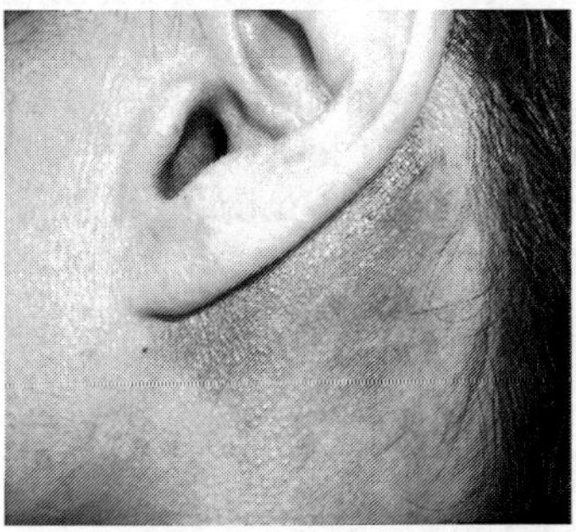

Explanation: Fracture of the temporal bone

The patient has a left postauricular ecchymosis, or Battle's sign, which can suggest underlying trauma to the temporal bone, as in this case. The patient had been intoxicated and recalled no trauma. Other signs of skull fracture include

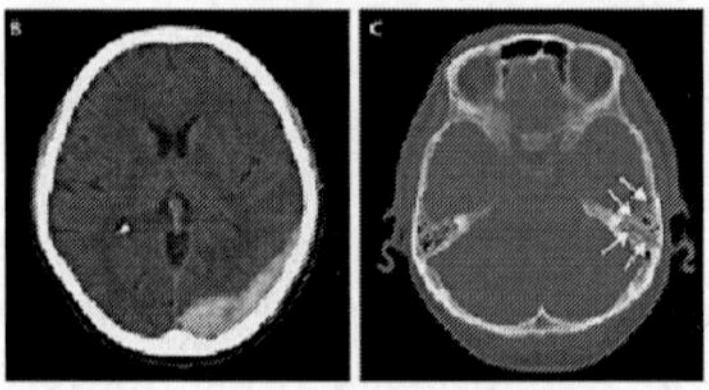

"raccoon eyes" when trauma involves the frontal bones of the skull.

Battle's sign represents ecchymosis around the mastoid process from head trauma that has caused a temporal bone fracture. The sign can suggest that a patient has sustained a significant blow to the skull, even if the medical history is obscure.

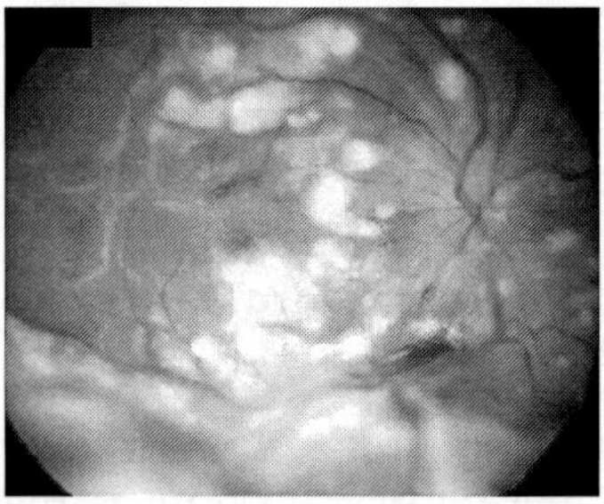

Explanation: Malignant hypertension

The retinal image demonstrates disk swelling with scattered cotton-wool spots, and inferior serous retinal detachment. The patient's blood pressure was 220/150 mm Hg. The pattern of subretinal fluid accumulation and exudative retinal detachment is most consistent with malignant hypertension.

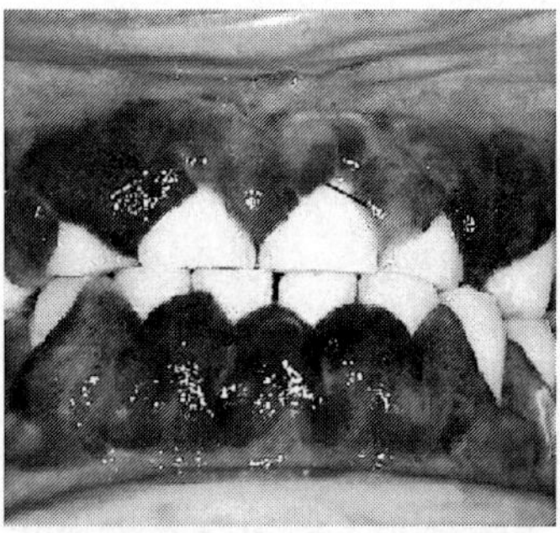

Explanation: Leukemia

Gingival infiltration in a patient with fever, fatigue, and weight loss is most suggestive of acute leukemia, especially monocytic variants of acute myelogenous leukemia. This patient's gingival infiltration resolved after treatment for acute myelomonocytic leukemia.

On physical examination, red, swollen gingivae, tender submandibular lymph nodes, and a palpable spleen were noted. Laboratory evaluation revealed a peripheral-blood white-cell count of 194,100 per cubic millimeter, with 44% blasts, and a peripheral-blood platelet count of 12,000 per cubic millimeter.

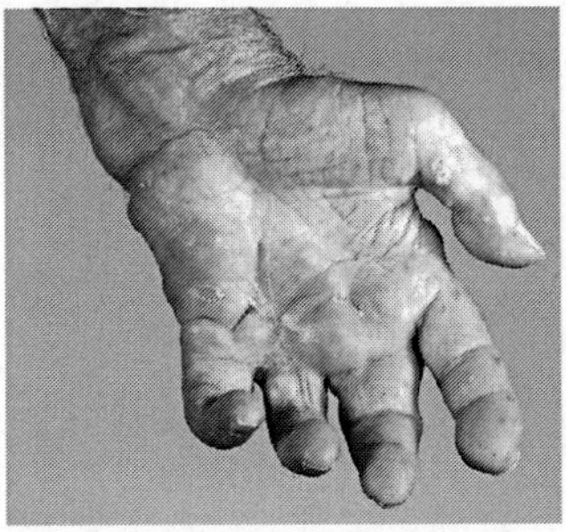

Explanation: Systemic sclerosis

Calcinosis cutis can be a complication of systemic sclerosis, the diagnosis in this case calcification of the skin is a feature of several connective tissue diseases. There is usually no detectable biochemical abnormality.

Widespread cutaneous calcification may be a feature of juvenile dermatomyositis. Usually there is an nonspecific illness with tender muscles. Once the diagnosis is made and corticosteroid therapy commenced there may be dramatic calcification.

Cutaneous calcification may be a feature of the CREST syndrome and Raynaud's disease. Calcium is deposited in the fingers and may discharge from the skin.

Bibliography

1. 10th Five Year Plan – Government of India, Planning Commission: Planning commission. nic.in/plans.planrel/fiv-eyr/welcome.html.
2. Adams O, Kinnon C. A Public Health Perspective. In UNCTADWHO Joint Publication, International Trade in Health Services: A Development Perspective, UNCTAD/ITCD/TSB/5–WHO/TFHE/98.1, Geneva, 1998.
3. Anand K, Chowdhury D, Singh KB, Pandav CS, Kapoor SK. Estimation of mortality and morbidity due to strokes in India. Neuroepidemiol 2001;20:208–11.
4. Assessing health needs. In: Wright J, Kyle D. Oxford Handbook of Public Health Practice, 2nd ed. 2007;20–31.
5. Assessing health status. In: Gentle P, Pencheon D, Flowers J (Eds). Oxford Handbook of Public Health Practice, 2nd ed. 2007;146–59.
6. Association of Schools of Public Health: www.asph.org
7. Bamji MS, Rao NP, Reddy V. Textbook of Human Nutrition, 2nd ed. New Delhi: Oxford & IBH Publishing Co Pvt Ltd, 2003.
8. Bedworth DA, Bedworth AE. Health education: A process for human effectiveness. New York: Harper and Row. 1978.
9. Beoglehole R, Bonita R. Public health at the cross-roads. Cambridge, UK:Cambridge University Press. 1997.
10. Berkson J. Limitation of the application of fourfold tables to hospital data. Biometrics Bull 1946;2:47–53.
11. Bertillon J. Classification of the causes of death (abstract). In: Transactions of the 15th International Congress on Hygiene Demography. Washington: 1912.
12. Bhatnagar D, Anand IS, Durrington PN, et al. Coronary risk factors in people from the Indian subcontinent living in west London and their siblings in India. Lancet 1995;345: 405–9.
13. Biostatistics Resources on the Web: www.sph.emory.edu/bios/bioslist.php
14. Breslow NE, Day NE. Statistical methods in cancer research. International Agency for Research on Cancer. Lyon;1980.
15. Bross IDJ. Determinacy of pertinancy of an extraneous variable. Jr chronic dis 1967;20:487–95.
16. Bunker JP. Improving Health: Measuring effects of medical care. Milbank quarterly. 1994;72:225–58.

17. Burbach HJ, Deker LE (Eds). A growing imperative. Planning and assessment in community education: Midland, Michigan, Pendell. 1977.
18. Buskirk ER, Iampietro PF, Bass DE. Work performance after dehydration: Effects of physical conditioning and heat acclimatization. J Appl Physiol 1958;12:189–94.
19. Cadarette BS, Sawka MN, Tover MM, Pandolf KB. Aerobic fitness and the hypohydration response to exercise-heat stress. Anat Space Environ Med 1984;14:194–8.
20. Caldwell CG, Kelley DB, Health CW. Jr Leukemia among Participants in Military Maneuvers at a Nuclear Bomb Test: A preliminary report. JAMA 1980;244:15754–8.
21. Cardiovascular Disease: WHO Publications :www.who.int/cardiovascular _ diseases/en/
22. CDC Cancer Prevention and Control: www.cdc.gov./cancer/index.htm
23. CDC: Disability and Health Team: www.cdc.gov/ncbddd/dh
24. CDC. Division of Violence Prevention: www.cdc.gov/ncipc
25. Census of India: www.censusindia.net/
26. Center for Science and Environment, India: www.cseindia.org
27. Central Pollution Control Board, India: www.epcb.nic.in
28. Chanda R. Trade in Health Services. ICRIER Working Paper No.70, Nov 2001.
29. Chaney MS, Ross ML. Nutrition. USA: Houghton Mifflin Company, 1996.
30. Choi BCK, Noseworthy AL. Classification, direction and prevention of bias in epidemiologic research. Jr Occup Med 1992;34:265–71.
31. Cholera: www.who.int/csr/resources/publications/cholera/
32. Ciminero AR, Calhoun KS, Adams HE (Eds). Handbook of behavioral assessment. New York, Wiley. 1977.
33. Climate and Health: Who www.who.int/mediacenter/factsheets/fs266/en/
34. Clinical Epidemiology Definitions: www.med.ualberta.ca/ebm/define.htm
35. Communication received from Mr. Ujjwal Kumar, WHO India office, 2006.
36. Cornfield J, Haenszel W, Hammord WC, Lukenfeld AM, Shimkin MB, Wyndea EC. Smoking and lung cancer: Recent evidence and a discussion of some questions. Jr Nat Cancer Instt 1959;22:173–203.
37. Criqvi MH, Austin M, Barrett Connor E. The effect of non-response on risk ratios in a cardiovascular disease study. Jr Chron Dis 1979;32:633–8.
38. Davidson S, Passmore R, Brock JF, Truswell AS. Human Nutrition and Dietetics, 6th ed. ELBS London: Churchill Livingstone 1975.

39. Department of public health. Georgia: Georgia Epidemiology Report. 1996;6.
40. Development of New Vaccines: www.who.int/mediacentre/factsheets/fs289/en/index.html
41. Dharmendra. Leprosy. 1st ed. Mumbai: Kothari Medical Publishing House. 1978;1.
42. Diabetes Mellitus: WHO: www.who.int/diabetes/facts/en/
43. Dignan MB, Carr PA. Introduction to program planning: A basic text for community health education. 1st ed. Philadelphia, Lea and Febiger. 1981.
44. Disabilities: World Health Organization: www.who.int/topics/disabilities/en/
45. Disability India: www.disabilityindia.org
46. Dr. (Brig) Sundarlal. Textbook of Community Medicine (PSM) CBS Publishers and Distributers, Delhi, 2002.
47. Dubos R. Man adapting. New haven, Yale Univ. 1965.
48. Engel GL. The need for a new medical model. A challenge for biomedicine. Science 1977;196:129.
49. Environmental Guidelines: India: www.ecoindia.com/ecobiz.htm
50. Environmental Health, WHO: www.who. int/topics/environmental_health/en/
51. Evans AS. Surveillance and seroepidemiology. Evans AS (Ed). In: Viral Infections of Humans. New York: Plenum Press. 1982:43–64.
52. Excite:Teaching Material for Epidemiology: www.cdc.gov/excite
53. Failure of extracranial-intracranial arterial bypass to reduce the risk of ischemic stroke. Results of an International Randomized Trial. New Eng J Med 1985;313:1191–200.
54. Family Welfare Program in India: mohfw.nic.in/dofw%20website family% 20welfare %20programme 5
55. Fox AJ, Colber PF. Low mortality rates in industrial cohort studies due to selection of work and survival in the industry. Brit J Prev Social Med 1976;30:225–30.
56. Gabr M. IUNS in the 21st century on the shoulders of 20th century giants of nutrition. In: Elmadfa I, Anklam E, Konig JS (Eds). Modern Aspects of Nutrition, Present Knowledge and Future Perspectives. 2003;56:13–8.
57. Gagge AP, Burlon AC, Bagett HC. A practical system for the description of heat exchange of man with his environment. Science 1941;94:928–30.
58. Ganapati R, Revankar CR. Leprosy. Quarterly Medical Review. 1992;44(1):1–3.
59. Gandy JW, Madden A, Holdsworth M. Oxford Handbook of Nutrition and Dietetics. New Delhi: Oxford University Press. 2007.
60. Gardner JW, Kark JA,Karnei K, et al. Risk factors predicting exertional heat illnesses in male Marine Corps recruits. Med Sci Sports Exerc 1996;28:939–44.

61. Garrow JS, James WPT, Ralph A. Human Nutrition and Dietetics. 10th ed. UK: Churchill Livingstone. 2000.
62. Geissler C, Powers H. Human Nutrition, 11th ed. London: Elsevier Churchill Livingstone. 2005.
63. Ghafoorunissa, Krishnaswamy K. Diet and Heart Disease. National Institute of Nutrition, Hyderabad, 2000.
64. Global Atlas of Infectious Diseases: Globalatlas.who.int/
65. Global Burden of Disease: www.who.int/evidence/bod
66. Global Fund for AIDS, TB and Malaria: www.globalfundatm.org/
67. Global warming: NASA maui.net~jstark/nasa.html
68. Global Water Supply and Sanitation Assessment Report 2000: www.who.int/water_sanitation_health/monitoring/jmp2000.pdf
69. Gopalan C, Ramasastri BV, Balasubramanium SC. Nutritive Value of Indian Foods, National Institute of Nutrition (ICMR), Hyderabad. 1999.
70. Government of India (ICMR and ICSSR). Health for all by the year 2000. An alternative strategy, 1980.
71. Government of India, Ministry of Health and FW. Report of a working group on health for all by the year 2000. New Delhi:1981.
72. Government of India. National Health Accounts: India, 2001–02, (New Delhi: Ministry of Health and Family Welfare, 2005).
73. Government of India. Report of the Committee on Multipurpose Workers Under Health and Family Planning Program, Department of Family Planning, Ministry of Health and Family Planning, New Delhi:1973.
74. Government of India. Report of the Health Survey and Development Committee. Simla: Govt of India Press, 1946.
75. Government of India. Report of the Health Survey and Planning Committee, Ministry of Health, Delhi:1962.
76. Government of India. Report of the National Commission on Macroeconomics and Health, 2006, Ministry of Health and Family Welfare.
77. Government of India, Report of the National Commission on Macroeconomics and Health. Ministry of Health and Family Welfare 2006.
78. Government of India. Swasth Hind, 1976.
79. Grant A. Laparoscopic compared with open methods of groin hernia repair: Systemic review of randomised controlled trial. Br J Surg 2006;87:860–7.
80. Green LW, Kreuter MW, Deeds SG, Partridge KB. Health Education Planning: A Diagnostic Approach. Palo Alto, Mayfield, 1980;86–115.
81. Groff JL, Gropper SS. Advanced Nutrition and Human Metabolism, 3rd ed. California: Wadsworth Thomson Learning. 2000.
82. Guidelines for Cholera Control. Geneva, WHO, 1993: www.who.int/csr/disease/cholera/ publications/en/

83. Guidelines of Biomedical Waste Management: India: www.epcb.nic.in/
84. Gupta R. Ghaffar A, Reddy KS, Singhi M. Rapid response to the burden of noncommunicable diseases in South Asia. 2004;328:807–10.
85. Gupta R. Trends in hypertension epidemiology in India. J Hum Hypertens 2004;18:73–8.
86. Hall TL, Mejia A (Eds). Principles, Methods, Issues. WHO, 1978.
87. Hamlin C, Sheard S. Revolutions in public health:1848 and 1998? BMJ 1998;317:587–91.
88. Hazards and Risk in the Workplace:www.agius.com/hew/resource/
89. Health aspects of air pollution: www.euro.who.int/document/E83080.pdf
90. Health care delivery: www.euro.who.int/eprise/main/who/Progs/Hcd/Home
91. Health economics: World Health Organization:www.who.int/topics/health-economics/en
92. Health Information of India,2007: cbhidghs.nic.in/hii2007/content1.asp
93. Health Policy and Planning: heapol.oupjournals.org
94. Horton R. The new public health of risk and radical engagement. Lancet 1998;352:251–2.
95. IMCI Information Package: www.who.int/child-adolescent-health/publications/IMCI/WHO_CHS_CAH _98.1HTM.
96. Immunization:www.who.int/mediacenter/factsheets/fs288/en/index.html
97. India Human Development Goals: www.undp.org.in/ihdg.htm.
98. Indicators of Child Health : www.who.int/child-adolescenthealth/OVER-VIEW/CHILD_HEALTH/child_monitoring.htm
99. Indoor Air Pollution and Health: www.who.int/ mediacentre/factsheets/fs292/en/index.html
100. Institute of Medicine, USA. The future of public health. Report of committee for the study of the future of public health. Washington, DC: National Academy Press. 1988;40–2. (Available at: http://fermat.nap.edu/catalog/1091 html (accessed in 2006).
101. International classification of diseases for oncology (ICD-O). 2nd ed. Geneva: World Health Organization. 1990.
102. International Classification of Functioning, Disability and Health: www.who.int/icf
103. International classification of impairments, disabilities and handicaps. A manual of classification relating to the consequences of disease. Geneva: World Health Organization. 1980.
104. International Diabetes Federation: www.idf.org/home/
105. International Labour Organization: Introduction to Occupational Health and Safety:www.itcilo.it/English/actrav/telearn/osh/intro/introduce.htm

106. International Plan of Action on Ageing, 2005: www. who.int/gb/ebwha/pdf_files/EB115/B115_29-en.pdf
107. International statistical classification of diseases and related health problems. Geneva: World Health Organization. 1993;1,2 and 3.
108. Jopling WF, Mc Dougall AC. Handbook of leprosy. 5th ed. Delhi: CBS Publishers. 1996.
109. Kark SL, Cobb S. From medicine in the community to community medicine. JAMA 1974;228:228.
110. Karon JM, Kupper LL. In defense of matching. Am J Epidemiol 1982;116:852–66.
111. Kearney PM, Whelton M, Reynolds K, Muntner P, Whelton PK, He J. Global burden of hypertension: Analysis of worldwide data. Lancet 2005;365:217–23.
112. Keith and Tone. Health Education. 2nd ed, Sylvia Tilfard. 1994.
113. Key Health Indicators, India 2007: cbhidghs.nic.in/indicate2007.HTM
114. King H, Aubert RE, Herman WH. Global burden of diabetes, 1995–2025: Prevalence, numerical estimates, and projections. Diabetes Care 1998;21:1414–31.
115. Kitagawa EM. Components of difference between two rates. Jr Am Stat Assn 1955;50:1168–94.
116. Klausen K, Dill DB, Phillips EE, McGregor D. Metabolic reactions to work in desert. J Appl Physiol 1967;22:292–6.
117. Kleiner SM. Nutrition guidelines for diet and health. In: Matzen RN and Lang RS (Eds): Clinical Preventive Medicine, 1st ed. USA: Mosby Publishers. 1993:385–410.
118. Klienbaum DG. Kupper LL, Morgenstern H. Epidemiologic research. Principles and quantitative methods. 1st ed. Van Nostrand Feinbold Company, New York.1982;40–61.
119. Klienbaum DG, Sullivan KM, Banker ND. Active Epi Companion Textbook. 1st ed. New York;Springer Verlag. 2000;17–35.
120. Kupper LL, Karon Jm, Khinbawn DG, Morgenstern H, Lewis DK. Matching in epidemiologic studies. Validity and efficiency considerations. Biometrics 1981;37:292–302.
121. Last JM. A dictionary of epidemiology. 2nd ed. New York: Oxford University Press.1988.
122. Leeder S, Raymond S, Greenberg H, Liu H, Esson K. A race against time. The challenge of cardiovascular disease in developing economies. New York: Columbia University. 2004.
123. Macroeconomics and Health: www.who.int/macrohealth/en/
124. Mahan LK, Stump SL. Krause's Food, Nutrition and diet therapy. 11th ed. Philadelphia, USA: Saunder's 2000.
125. Malaria: www.who.int/mediacenter/factsheets/fs094/en/
126. Managing an outbreak of acute diarrhea: www.who.int/csr/resources/publications/cholera/WHOCDSCSRNCS20037.pdf

127. Mandel E. Health Promotion. USA:Elsevier, 2006.
128. Masi AT. Potential uses and limitations of hospital data in epidemiologic research. Am J Pub Health 1965;55:658–67.
129. Maternal and Newborn Health: www.who.int/reproductive-health/MNBH/index.htm
130. Mc Collum EV. A history of nutrition, Boston. Houghton Miffin Company, 1957.
131. McKeigue PM, Miller GJ, Marmot MG. Coronary heart disease in South Asians overseas: A review. J Clin Epidemiol 1989;42:597–609.
132. Measuring health needs. In: Mooney G, Jan S, Wishman V. Oxford Textbook of Public Health, 4th ed. 2002;1765–72.
133. Mehta SR, Jaswal DS. Heat stroke. MJAFI 2003;59:140–3.
134. Millennium development goals: A compact among nations to end poverty. Human Development Report 2003. UNDP.
135. Millennium Development Goals: www.undp.org/mdg/
136. Miller LK. Principles of everyday behavior analysis. Monterey, California. Brooks-Cole, 1975.
137. Ministry of Environment and Forests, India: envfor.nic.in
138. Ministry of Health and Family Welfare,India: www.mohfw.nic.in
139. Ministry of Social Welfare, Delhi: www.socialwelfare.delhigovt.nic.in
140. Mohan V, Shanthirani S, Deepa R, Premalatha G, Sastry NG, Saroja R. Intra-urban differences in the prevalence of the metabolic syndrome in southern India—The Chennai Urban Population Study (CUPS No. 4). Diabet Med 2001;18: 280–7.
141. Murray CJL, Lopez AD. Global health statistics. Global burden of disease and injury series. Boston MA: Harvard School of Public Health. 1996.
142. Mustard HS, Stebbins EC. An introduction to public health. 4th ed. New York: Macmillan. 1959.
143. Nandraj S, Duggal S. Physical Standards in the Private Health Sector. http://www.cehat.org/publications/pb10a53.htm
144. National AIDS Control Organization: www.nacoonline.org
145. National Cancer Registry Programme. Two year report of the population-based cancer registries 1997–1998. Incidence and distribution of cancer. New Delhi: Indian Council of Medical Research. 2002.
146. National Health Profile 2007. Central Bureau of Health Intelligence, Government of India, Director General of Health Services. New Delhi.
147. National Health Profile. Central Bureau of Health Intelligence, Government of India, Director General Health Services, New Delhi:2007.
148. National Institute of Mental Health. USA: www.nimh.nih.gov
149. National Institute on Aging: www.nia.nih.gov

150. National Leprosy Eradication Program, India: mohfw.nic.in/nlep.htm
151. National Population Policy: mohfw.nic.in/dofw%20 website/national%20population%20policy/npp.htm
152. National Program for Control of Blindness and Eye Awarness: mohfw.nic.in/index.htm#NPCB
153. National Rural Health Mission: mohfw.nic.in
154. Neyman J. Statistics-servant of all services. Science 1955;122:401.
155. Nick Drager and David P. Fidler, GATS and Health Related Services: Managing Liberalization of Trade in Service from a Health Policy Perspective. WHO, 2004.
156. NIOSH:Occupational Diseases–A Guide to Their Recognition: www.cdc.gov/niosh/77-181.html
157. Obesity and Overweight: WHO: www.who.int/hpr/nph/docs/gs_obesity.pdf
158. Overweight and Obesity: CDC: www.cdc.gov/nccdphp/dnpa/obesity/index.htm
159. Pandolf KB, Griffin TB, Munro EN, Goldman RF. Heat intolerance as a function of percent of body surface involved with Miliaria rubra. Am J Physiol 1980;239:R233–40.
160. Park K. Epidemiology of communicable diseases: Textbook of Preventive and Social Medicine, 19th ed. Jabalpur: Banarsidas Bhanot Publishers. 2007.
161. Pasricha S. Count what you eat. National Institute of Nutrition ICMR Hyderabad:1989.
162. Patel JV, Vyas A, Cruickshank JK, et al. Impact of migration on coronary heart disease risk factors: Comparison of Gujaratis in Britain and their contemporaries in villages of origin in India. Atherosclerosis 2005.
163. Paukin DM, Muir CS, Whelan SL, Gao YT, Ferlay J, Powell J (Eds). Cancer incidence in five continents. Lyon, France:IARC Scientific Publication. 1992;6.
164. Peterson DR. The clinical study of social behavior. New York: Appleton- Century-Crofts. 1968.
165. Pneumoconioses: www.cdc.gov/niosh/topics/pneumoconioses/
166. Prabhakaran GN. National Health Reports. In: Policies and Program Health in India. New Delhi: Jaypee Brothers Medical Publishers (P) Ltd. 2005.
167. Prentice RL, Kakar F, Hursting S, et al. Aspects of rationale for women's health trial. J National Cancer Instt 1988;80:802–14.
168. Preventing Emerging Infectious Diseases: www.cdc.gov/ncidod/emergplan/index.htm
169. Ramachandran A. Epidemiology of diabetes in India—Three decades of research. India: J Assoc Physicians 2005;53:34–8.
170. Reddy KS. Cardiovascular disease in India. World Health Stat Q 1993;46:101–7.

171. Reddy KS, Gupta PC (Eds). Tobacco Control in India. New Delhi: Ministry of Health and Family Welfare, Government of India. 2004.
172. Registrar General of India. Census 2001.
173. Rehabilitation Council of India: www.rehabcouncil.nic.in
174. Report of the Working Group on Integrating Nutrition with Health for the XI Five Year Plan (2007–2012 Government of India. Ministry of Women and Child Development, Nov 2006.
175. Reproductive Health Library: www.who.int/reproductie-health/rhl/index.html
176. Richardson BW. The health of nations: A review of the works of Edwin Chadwick. London: Longmans, Green and Co. 1887;2.
177. Roberts RS, Spitzer WO, Delmore T, Sackett DL. An empirical demonstration of Berksons Bias. Jr Chron Dis 1978;31: 119–28.
178. Roll Back Malaria Partnership: rbm.who.int/cgi/bin/rbm/rbmportal/custom/rbm/home.do
179. Rose SD. A casebook in group therapy: A behavioral cognitive approach. Englewood Cliffs, Prentice Hall, 1980.
180. Rossi PH, Freemen HE, Wright SR. Evaluation: A systemic approach. Beverly Hills, Sage. 1979.
181. Rowell LB, Brengelmann GL, Murray JA, Kraning KK, Kusumi F. Human metabolic responses to hyperthermia during mild to maximal exercise. J Appl Physiol 1969;26:395–402.
182. Rubin DR. Matching to remove bias in observational studies. Biometrics 1973;29:159–83.
183. Sacket DL. Bias in analytical research. Jr Chronic Dis 1979; 32:51–63.
184. Sacket DL. Bias in analytical research. Jr Chronic Dis 1979;32:51–63.
185. Sartwell PE. Retrospective studies: A review for the clinician. Ann Intern Med 1974;81:381–6.
186. Sawka MN, Toner MM, Francesconi RP, Pandolf KB. Hypohydration and exercise: Effects of heat acclimation, gender and environment. J Appl Physiol 1983;55:1147–53.
187. Shattuck L. Report of the sanitary commission of Massachusetts, 1850. (Dutton and Westworth, state Printers, Boston, 1850). Cambridge: Harvard University Press. 1948.
188. Sheps CG. Milbank Memorial Fund Commission Report: Human education and public health. New York: Prodist. 1976.
189. Sigerist HE. A history of medicine. Preventive and Archaic Medicine. New York:Oxford University Press; 1951;1.
190. Soanes C. Oxford Dictionary. Oxford: 9th ed. Oxford University Press, 2001.
191. Sriramachari S. Heat hyperpyrexia: Time to act. Indian J Med Res 2004;119:7–10.
192. Srivastava A, Pal H, Dwivedi SN, Pandey A, Pande JN. National household survey of drug and alcohol abuse in India. Report

accepted by the Ministry of Social Justice and Empowerment, Government of India and UN Office or Drug and Crime, Regional Office of South Asia, New Delhi. 2004

193. Staci N. Williams Basic Nutrition and Diet Therapy, 12th ed. USA. Mosby, Elsevier. Missouri:2005.
194. Surveillance of risk factors for noncommunicable diseases. The WHO STEP wise approach. Noncommunicable diseases and mental health. Geneva: World Health Organization. 2003;18. International Institute for Population Sciences. National Family Health Survey. 1998–99 (NFHS – 2) Mumbai: IIPS 2000.
195. Susser MW, Watson W. Sociology in Medicine. London: Oxford University Press, 1971.
196. The Global Polio Eradication Initiative: www.polioeradication.org/
197. The ICD-10 classification of mental and behavioral disorders: Clinical descriptions and diagnostic guidelines. Geneva: World Health Organization, 1992.
198. The Stop Tuberculosis Initiative Website: www.stoptb.org/
199. Todd WTA, Lockwood DNJ, Sundar S (Eds). Infectious diseases. Davidson's Principles and Practise of Medicine, 20th ed. Churchill Livingstone Publications, Elsevier. 2006.
200. Todhunter EN. Chronology of some events in the development and application of the science of nutrition. Nutrition Reviews 1976;34:354–75.
201. Tuberculosis Control: India: www.tbcindia.org/documents.asp
202. Tuberculosis Research Center, Chennai: www.trc-chennai.org /
203. UNAIDS India: www.unaids.org.in
204. United States Department of Health Education and Welfare. Techniques of vital statistics 1965. Vital statistics rates in the United States 1900–40. Washington DC. NATIONAL CENTER FOR HEALTH STATISTICS.
205. USDHEW, PHS, HRA. Educating the public about health: A planning guide. Washington, HEW publication No. (HRA)-78–14004, Oct 1977.
206. US Health and Human Services, Public Health Service. For a healthy nation: Returns on investment in public health. Washington. DC:US Government Printing Office, 1995.
207. US Public Health Service. For a healthy nation: Returns on investments in public health. Washington, DC:US Government Printing Office. 1994;42.
208. Vaccine development and control of communicable diseases: www.wpro.who.int/rcm/en/archives/rc39/wpr-rc39r11.htm
209. Vatsyanan. Principles of Sociology. Publishers: Kedarnath, Ramnath, Meerut (India).

210. Vaugham JP, Morrow RH. Manual of Epidemiology for District Health Management. 1st ed. World Health Organization, Geneva. 1989:15–6.
211. Waste Management: WHO: www.who.int/topics/waste_management/en/
212. Water and Sanitation Program: www.wsp.org/
213. Water in India: www.devalt.org/water/waterinindia.htm3.9
214. Weiss CH. Evaluation research: Methods and assessing program effectiveness. Englewood Cliffs, Prentice Hall. 1972.
215. White C. Research on smoking and lung cancer: A landmark in the history of chronic disease epidemiology. Yale Jr of bio med1990;63:29–46.
216. WHO Cancer Control Program: www.who.int/cancer/en
217. WHO.Department of Injury and Violence Prevention: www.who.int/violence_injury_prevention/en
218. WHO Guidelines on Hypertension: www.who.int/cardiovascular_diseases/ guidelines/hypertension_guidelines.
219. WHO's Global TB Program : www.who.ch/gtb
220. WHO Statistical Resources: www.who.int/emcdocuments/surveillance/does/whocdscrisr992ann.pdf.
221. WHO: Water, Sanitation and Health: www.who.int/water_sanitation_health/en/
222. Winslow CEA. The untilled fields of public health, Science 1920;51:23.
223. Workplace Safety and Health: www.cdc.gov/node.do/id/0900f3ec8000ec09
224. World Bank. Human Resources for Health Policies: A Critical Component in Health Policies, HNP Discussion Paper, 2004.
225. World Health Organization: Aging: www.who.int/topics/ageing/en/
226. World Health Organization. A guide to eliminating leprosy as a public health problem. Geneva:WHO. 1982.
227. World Health Organization Alcohol Abuse and Alcoholism: www.who.int/substance-abuse
228. World Health Organization. Energy and protein requirements. Technical Report Series No. 724. Geneva:1985.
229. World Health Organization. Measuring the levels of health: Report of a study group. WHO TRS 1957;137.
230. World Health Organization: Task Force on Health Economics: www.who.int/medicine/library/edu-general/who-tfhe-97-1
231. World Health Organization. Tech Rep Ser No 675. Geneva:WHO. 1982.
232. World Health Organization. Tech Rep Ser No 874 (WHO expert committee on leprosy). Geneva:WHO. 1998.

233. World Health Organization. The Constitution of World Health Organization. WHO Chron 1947;1:29.
234. World Health Organization. Weekly Epidemiological Record No 20, 2001.
235. World Health Organization. Weekly Epidemiological Record No 28, 2000.
236. World Health Organization. Weekly Epidemiological Record No 33, 2008.
237. World Health Organization. Weekly Epidemiological Record No 20–1,1994.
238. World Health Organization. Weekly Epidemiological Record No 31, 2006.
239. World Health Organization (WHO). Geneva: Health for All Series, Serial no. 1–8.
240. World Health OrganizationWHO. www.who.int/topics/occupational_health/en/
241. World Health Report: Statistical Annex: www. who.int/shr/2004/annex/en/index.html
242. World Report:Road Traffic Injury Prevention: www.who.int/world-health-ay/2004/informaterials/world_report/en/index.html
243. WTO, Health and Social Services: Background Note by the Secretariat, 18 Sept 1998, paragraph4,http://www.wto.org/english/tratop_e/serv_e/health_social_e/health_social_e.htm (visited 17 Aug 2006).
244. Wyndham CH. Research in the human sciences in the gold mining industries. Amer Indust Hyg Assoc J 1947;35:113–36.
245. Yusuf S, Hawken S, Ounpuu S, et al. Effect of potentially modifiable risk factors associated with myocardial infarction in 52 countries (the INTERHEART study): Case-control study. Lancet 2004;364:937–52.
246. Zoonoses: www.int/zoonoses/en/